NO TIME FOR JELLO

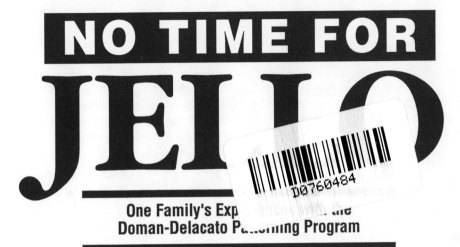

One Family's Experience with the Doman-Delacato Patterning Program

By Berneen Bratt

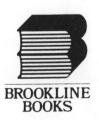

BROOKLINE BOOKS

Copyright © 1989 by Berneen Bratt

Library of Congress Cataloging-in-Publication Data

Bratt, Berneen. 1947-
　　No time for jello / by Berneen Bratt.
　　　　p.　　cm.
　　Bibliography: p.
　　ISBN 0-914797-56-5
　　1. Cerebral palsied children—Rehabilitation. I. Title
RJ496.C4B69 1989
618.92'836—dc19　　　　　　　　　　　　　　　　　89-781
　　　　　　　　　　　　　　　　　　　　　　　　　　　　CIP

Published by
Brookline Books, Inc.
PO Box 1046
Cambridge, MA 02238-1046

Printed in the United States of America.

To my dad,
Barnard G. Mallard

Thanks for the love and strength

Preface

Albert Einstein once said that, in spite of everything else, remember your humanity. Coming from a man immersed in both scientific and humanitarian affairs, such a sentiment is perhaps not surprising, but it is noteworthy as an admonition that science cannot be divorced from human affairs.

I am reminded of this statement in reading Berneen Bratt's book on her and her family's experiences in the patterning program of the Institutes for the Achievement of Human Potential (IAHP). Up until now, the debate as to the effectiveness of the Doman-Delacato "patterning" techniques has for the most part followed the classic scientific progression: one side presents what appears a startling new advance or cure, the other examines the evidence and points out either logical or methodological flaws. Advocates then produce counterclaims, which are in turn counter-counterclaimed. To the outsider not involved in the debate, the whole process seems esoteric, sterile, . . . and even a little unreal.

Begun almost 30 years ago, the entire debate over the Doman-Delacato therapies has generally followed this progression. Based on late-19th century ideas of evolutionary theory and studies purporting to show that the procedures cause dramatic improvements in children with handicapping conditions, the patterning procedures were first thought to be a "new hope for brain-damaged children" (see Warshaw, 1982 for a review of accounts in the popular press). IAHP personnel wrote books and scientific articles to substantiate their claims and a spate of laudatory articles followed in the popular press. Was this really a "cure" for mental retardation, cerebral palsy, or other debilitating conditions?

The answer, at least to most professionals, is no. The theoretical underpinnings of the procedures—Haeckel's recapitulationist theory—seem disproven, as "the history of biology is replete with considerations of the weakness of recapitulationist theory and no substantial support for the general viewpoint can be drawn from current consideration of the nervous system and its development" (Cohen, Birch, & Taft, 1970, p. 162). Similarly, the studies of dramatic improvements appear, upon closer inspection, to be unsupported (see Zigler & Hodapp, 1986, Ch. 8). When careful studies have been performed, little or no improvements in children's functioning have been demonstrated, leading to the disavowal of these procedures by the American Academy of Pediatrics and other groups interested in retarded children.

But such scientific critiques, while important, are unable to show the human side of the issue. It is this human side that comes through so clearly in the book before you.

Berneen Bratt's book is a quest: a quest for the best for her child with cerebral palsy and a quest for knowledge. On one level, it is a simple, straightforward tale showing a family's involvement in a cure for their boy's problems. Mrs. Bratt takes us from Jamie's birth, to early suspicions that there are problems, to encounters with medical and school professionals—the common, if lamentable, experiences of parents with a handicapped child.

But the experiences of the Bratt family go beyond the ordinary in that they succumb to a costly, time-consuming, and—to most professionals—an ineffective therapy. Mrs. Bratt shows this therapy in action, from the IAHP talks in Philadelphia to the daily therapeutic grind of moving Jamie's arms one way X number of times, to making him do Y amount of crawling, etc. The reader comes to *know* what the patterning therapy is about—in a way simply not expressible in standard scientific writing.

On another level, however, the story in *No Time for Jello* is more than a description of either the Bratt family or their involvement in the IAHP therapy. It is a cautionary tale showing how and why a middle-class, educated family could fall victim to a therapy that doesn't work. The patina of scientism—the allure of the seemingly scientific—can override skepticism of even the most knowledgeable individuals. In addition, the book powerfully evokes the emotional ups and downs associated with any therapy. Parents first feel extremely good about finally finding something that seems to work, that is finally able to help their disabled child. Later, however, ineffective therapies become suspect, as the parent sees that—no matter what anyone says—the promised changes are simply not occurring. The issue then becomes how to get off of what has become an emotional roller coaster.

Mrs. Bratt got off her roller coaster by withdrawing from the IAHP therapies and by writing this book. She learned more about the procedures and more about why the majority of professionals do not advocate these techniques. It is not, as IAHP personnel claim, that professionals "don't care," or that they are "out to get the IAHP," but because the therapy does not seem to work. As we conclude in our recent book, "there does not appear to be any justification for [the IAHP therapies's] continued use" (Zigler & Hodapp, 1986, p. 191; see also Spitz, 1986). Mrs. Bratt knows this, in a way and with a degree of conviction that reading this book with reveal. We can only thank and commend her for a courageous act, as she has produced a clear, simple, yet powerful work that joins science and humanity.

Edward Zigler
Sterling Professor of Psychology
Yale University
Jan. 17, 1989

REFERENCES

Cohen, H.J., Birch, H.B., & Taft, L.T. (1970). Some considerations for evaluating the Doman-Delacato patterning method. *Pediatrics, 45,* 302-314.

Spitz, H. (1986). *The raising of intelligence: A selected history of attempts to raise retarded intelligence.* Hillsdale, NJ: Lawrence Erlbaum.

Warshaw, R. (1982). The minds of children. *Philadelphia Magazine,* April, 120-124; 180-189.

Zigler, E. & Hodapp, R.M. (1986). *Understanding mental retardation.* New York: Cambridge University Press.

Table of Contents

Part III: After the Program

Introduction

Pearl S. Buck wrote more than 30 years ago in her book *The Child Who Never Grew* that because parents of brain injured children are

> ...driven by the conviction that there must be someone who can cure, we take our children over the surface of the whole earth, seeking the one who can heal. We spend all the money we have and we borrow until there is no one else to lend. We go to doctors good and bad, to anyone, for only a wisp of hope. We are gouged by unscrupulous men who make money from our terror, but now and again we meet those saints who, seeing the terror and guessing the empty purse, will take nothing for their advice, since they cannot heal (p. 17).

No Time for Jello: One Family's Experience With Patterning is the story of my family's search for help for our brain injured child. Our journey led us down different paths and decisions than did Pearl Buck's journey. And we met none of the saints to whom she refers.

Moreover, this book is the story of my family's experiences with the controversial therapy, called "patterning," prescribed by the Institutes for Achievement of Human Potential in Philadelphia. I hope that my description of the theory and techniques of the Institutes, and of our personal recovery, will be educative to both professionals and families.

Berneen Bratt
May 1986

PART I

BEFORE THE PROGRAM

1
The Beginning

I looked up just in time to see the streaker run across the stage.

It was after one a.m. and I was unusually tired. I had only intended to open my eyes briefly, in order to see what exotic gown Elizabeth Taylor might be wearing. But thanks to the six inch Sony, neither gown nor streaker could be seen in much detail. No matter. My greater interest was in the reactions of the celebrities at the Academy Awards Ceremony. I imagined that millions of other television viewers around the world, who, like me, had endured hours of lesser awards in anticipation of the greater awards, had now, also like me, ceased their dozing, and were suddenly watching and listening with renewed enthusiasm.

I shifted my position in my hospital bed, and leaned forward to turn up the volume on the tiny TV. I was careful not to disturb my newborn son nursing at my breast.

Elizabeth Taylor and David Niven had been about to present the final award for the best movie of the year. When the laughter and surprised exclamations from the audience of stars tapered off, Elizabeth Taylor said, "That's a pretty hard act to follow." and David Niven, with his usual cool reserve, observed, "That's probably the only laugh that man will ever get in his life—stripping off his clothes and showing us his shortcomings."

The most eagerly awaited award would be less well remembered by the public than the unprecedented event that had occurred just prior to its presentation. The ripped envelope revealed that the best movie of 1973 was *The Sting*.

Alden and I had arrived at the hospital around eight a.m. on a sunny cold day, the 28th of March. I had been in mild labor for several hours at home. In the labor room, I donned a hospital johnny and submitted to all the routine preparations for delivery. The nurse took my blood pressure four times in a matter of minutes. Then my obstetrician came in to personally read my blood pressure. That seemed unusual.

"Your blood pressure is very high. 140/100." It was usually around 110/70. "You're not dilated much so it will be a long wait for delivery. We need to give you something to bring down that pressure to protect you and the baby."

The doctor had a soft, calm voice. I agreed to the medication. I hadn't taken any medication throughout my pregnancy until January. Then my doctor had prescribed a diuretic because I was so swollen with retained fluid. I took that for the last trimester. And for the last two weeks I had been taking an antibiotic and a decongestant for a flu-like illness. I had been bedridden and had eaten poorly during that time.

Soon Alden came into the labor room with me. He was a handsome, curly-haired, full-blood Swede who resembled a short Ted Kennedy and was still asked for his ID at 37. The doctor told Alden not to worry about my blood pressure, so we relaxed and talked about the breathing exercises we had learned to do in our natural childbirth classes. As many couples were doing at this time, we were going to have this baby together and with as little medication as possible.

During the next few hours, I was drowsy and I remembered a nurse giving me more pills and shots and taking my blood pressure. I longed for this part to be over. I awoke around two-thirty. Alden and my doctor were standing over me.

"We have to do a Caesarean, Berneen. You have toxemia and you and the baby may be in danger if we wait any longer." I was stunned. What kind of danger? What had changed to make them decide to do it now and not two hours earlier? But there wasn't time for any further conversation. They were definitely in a hurry.

Later I learned that because of my elevated blood pressure and the analysis of my blood and urine, I was considered to be severely preeclamptic. (Eclampsia is a major cause of toxemia of pregnancy, possibly leading to convulsions, coma, or death.) My symptoms were not responding well to medical management and my labor was questionable. Delivery of the infant was the one remedy left for my condition.

I was wheeled out of the labor room toward an elevator that would take me down to the operating room. Alden kissed me at the door to the elevator and tried to be reassuring.

"See you soon, Mommy."

Fathers were not allowed in the operating room in 1974. As he went off to the waiting room, I wondered what his blood pressure was. Things were not going quite as well as we had planned.

I don't remember anything until the next morning. Alden came in. He told me we had a baby boy. That was the first mention of our baby I'd heard. I couldn't stay awake, but I went back to sleep happy.

By the next afternoon, I was fully awake and aware. It was almost 48 hours after the birth of our son Jamieson Alden. I was out of danger and I was told that our baby was doing fine. A nurse brought him to me, and I held him a long time that first time. He was six pounds, thirteen ounces, had a full head of dark hair, and looked exactly like his father.

Jamie had remained in an isolette for close observation since birth, because he was not as pink as he should be. On Tuesday morning I made my first stroll down the hall. It was also Jamie's first day out of the isolette and in the regular nursery with the other babies. My doctor said that I would be able to go home on Thursday, but the pediatrician said that Jamie could not go home until he maintained or gained weight. He was the right color now, but he was still losing weight. I hoped at every feeding on Tuesday and Wednesday that he would gain. On Thursday morning he had gained one half ounce. So on the seventh day, a sunny April morning, Alden and I brought our perfect little Jamieson Alden Bratt home to Kittery, Maine.

Our birth announcement accurately expressed how we felt. On the outside it said, "We are no longer the happiest couple in town"; on the inside it said, "Now we are the happiest family in town."

Jamie and I spent a leisurely summer playing, visiting with my closest friend Susan Berry in Massachusetts, and going to the beach as often as possible. He was extremely good natured, had a winning smile, and was obviously intelligent, sensitive, and observant. He got much attention from strangers whenever I took him anywhere. A woman in a department store once said, "Why, his eyes look like two big blueberries!"

But two small things about Jamie began to concern me. I noticed early in the summer that he kept his head turned to the far right. It did not seem to hurt him if I manually turned his head to the left while he was sleeping or sitting, but he would turn back as soon as I let go. I tried to have people and other interesting things to his left, but he would still look at the blank wall on his right.

Later in the summer, when Jamie began to reach for objects, he never reached with his right hand. His left hand shot out eagerly for anything that looked inviting, while the right hand remained immobile. I was not at all opposed to my son being left-handed. It just bothered me that I couldn't entice him to use his right hand at all.

I watched him for several weeks to be sure they persisted. At Jamie's six-month check-up, the pediatrician said that for the last few weeks in utero a baby is obliged to keep his head sideways as he becomes more crowded. Jamie had obviously kept his head turned to the right inside of me. As for the hand, that was just early handedness preference. The doctor dangled some plastic keys over Jamie and when he grabbed them with his left hand, the doctor said, "Yep, he's going to be a lefty."

I was initially relieved by these simple explanations. But as the weeks passed, the fears about Jamie's neck and hand crept back. Why couldn't Jamie sit up alone or stand or creep yet? He was physically active but lacked the coordination and balance to sit, stand, and crawl. When I placed him in a sitting position, he would catch himself when he tipped to the left, but when he leaned to the right, he would fall over. When I stood him at the coffee table, he held on so tightly with his left hand that the fingers turned white, and would finally fall down. He did wiggle his right arm, in a random, uncontrolled manner, but mostly he held it stiffly, turned slightly inward, with a tight fist. Normally a child at that age would use two hands to hold onto a toy or to transfer it from one hand to the other as part of exploration. Jamie never did this. In the tub he splashed vigorously with all limbs—except his right arm.

It also seemed that his use of his right leg was limited. He never supported any of his weight on that leg to stand. When he took steps while holding my hands, he got off his right leg quickly. It was not as stiff as the arm, but it was definitely not normal.

At almost eight months old, my baby could not do much but lay around on the floor. Slowly, this realization came over me, and it was numbing. I had spent a lot of time hoping what I saw would go away. Some people told me that just because I used to teach disabled children I was looking too hard at my son's development and trying to find something wrong. Or that one side was just developing more slowly. I knew that development proceeded symmetrically and there should be no lag on one side.

We needed to take Jamie to a doctor. But who? I surely was not going to go to our old pediatrician to hear more nonsense about what side Jamie had lain on inside me or that handedness could be determined so early.

In November I took Jamie to an orthopedic surgeon. The doctor had a cool, aloof manner as he asked me the routine questions about delivery and milestones. He took X-rays of Jamie's arm and leg to rule out any bone abnormalities. He examined Jamie briefly and wiggled the arm a little. Then he told me to exercise the arm and come back in six months. I went home feeling confused. I had no definite diagnosis and no definite treatment.

In December I took Jamie to yet another doctor. This time I was extremely impressed. He was thorough in his questions and in his examination of Jamie. I got the feeling that he had a good idea of what Jamie could and could not do with that arm. During that visit he called the birth defects clinic at a major hospital in Boston and made appointments for Jamie to see three specialists in January. I knew we were going to settle this once and for all, and at a place where I could feel confident.

Our first appointment at the Boston hospital was at ten-thirty, and we arrived with time to spare. We found ourselves in a large waiting room, filled with parents and children of all ages, and varying mental and physical disabilities. Jamie was content to sit quietly on my lap. He stared openly at the people around us; Alden and I stared on the sly. One child was banging his head methodically on the floor in front of us, two more were slumped in child-sized wheelchairs. Many were in immobile heaps on the floor.

We were called to an examining room and met the doctor who was to be our coordinator. She examined him thoroughly, finally provoking him to tears. She noted that his head tilted to the right, that there was too much tone in the arm and too little tone in the leg. She suspected a possible pinched nerve or missing vertebra in the spine and sent us upstairs for X-rays. She handed us his folder and asked us to return it to her at the end of the day.

We went to the X-ray department and found they did not allow a parent to accompany a child. Jamie, along with the X-ray, was plunked back in my lap 15 minutes later, sobbing pathetically, his clothes on crooked, having endured his second ordeal of the day. He recovered as I sat on the floor and fed him his lunch.

The orthopedic surgeon, in another building, was quicker in his examination and didn't offer any conclusions, saying he would call the first doctor.

While waiting for the third doctor, a pediatric neurologist, I began to leaf through Jamie's folder. There were pages and pages of nurses' notes from the hospital where Jamie was born. The observations told of "duskiness... tremors lasting several seconds...sleepy most of the time...fixed stare...rigidity," and on and on. Once a doctor had been summoned for Jamie in the middle of the night because he was believed to be in some sort of danger. We hadn't been informed of any of this.

Jamie's pediatrician had glossed over the reasons he had been kept in an isolette for four days after birth, and had ignored my later concerns that there might be something wrong with Jamie. Surely the doctor knew that these observations, coupled with the circumstances of my baby's birth, made my child at high risk for sustaining some sort of birth defect. Why hadn't he been honest with me? I had known that something was wrong with Jamie in the first weeks of his life, and yet my pediatrician had denied it, treating me as an inexperienced, overreacting mother.

Dread replaced my initial feeling of anger, and tears blurred the words. I understood why I was at one of the most advanced medical centers in the world.

The neurologist didn't even want to look at the X-rays. He knew they would not show what he knew to be present in Jamie's brain: lesions indicating nerve damage on the left side of the brain, causing difficulty on the whole right side of the body. Because of my high blood pressure during labor, he explained that Jamie had experienced, probably shortly before birth, what would be similar to a stroke in an elderly patient. One or more blood vessels in his brain had burst, the deprived brain cells had died, and whatever functions those cells had controlled were lost or impaired forever. When this happens to an infant, the child can possibly recover some functions more easily than when this happens to an adult. For example, the speech center, normally on the left side of the brain, had probably already switched over to the right side, as Jamie seemed to be developing reasonably well in that area. Cerebral palsy, or CP, is a catch-all term for people with this type of brain damage.

The doctor assured us that I had good prenatal care and that things were done properly at delivery. It just happened sometimes under my particular set of circumstances. He said that Jamie might or might not have difficulty walking normally, and if he did have problems, the orthopedic man we had seen would help. He said that Jamie would never have full use of his right hand, but exactly how limited he would be was hard to tell right now. And he said that his right arm and leg would be slightly smaller than the left arm and leg. Furthermore, he warned that any person who had suffered brain damage was a likely candidate for seizures or a learning disability, and when Jamie was three or four, one or the other might show up.

It was his opinion that Jamie was intellectually "up to snuff," and that in ten years we could expect to have a very handsome boy, doing well in school, with only a minor physical problem, and, perhaps, a learning disability. Meanwhile, we should exercise his limbs three times a day for 10 minutes at a time, to prevent them from stiffening or atrophying due to nonuse. Then, when he was old enough, Jamie could make them move himself to continue his exercises. There were some cases of cerebral palsy that benefitted from surgery that moved muscles around, and other cases that responded well to medication to relax the muscles. The neurologist did not recommend either of these treatments for Jamie at this time.

During the short revisit with our coordinator, we learned that they would like to see Jamie every six months to evaluate his progress and make new treatment recommendations as needed. There would be no charge for these future visits since a federal grant and the March of Dimes covered such expenses.

As we began our drive home, Jamie finally got to take a long overdue nap in his car seat, and I sat gloomily in the front seat. It had taken more than nine months of worry and chasing around to find out the truth. Now that we knew what had happened in the past and what we could expect for the present, we still didn't know what the future would hold for Jamie.

Alden reached over to hold my hand. He said, "We know he won't be a watchmaker or a right-handed pitcher for the Red Sox, but I think he'll do all right. We'll help him overcome his difficulties as they arise."

I thought about what Jamie's difficulties might be. How would he ever be able to tie his shoes, cut his meat, zip his jacket, climb a tree, ride a bike, drive a car, play baseball, swim, ski, or golf? The list was endless and the answers unbearable. It was a two-handed world. I closed my eyes in despair and napped along with Jamie.

2

Birth Defects Are Forever

Jamie could now sit alone and walk very well holding my two hands. It was a nuisance because that was all he wanted to do every waking hour. He was very demanding about it, and screeched if someone, preferably me, didn't walk him when he wanted to walk. Sometimes he even ran. I was becoming a hunchback. Alden could hardly do it because of his severely arthritic right hip, but he did it every day when he came home from work. Jamie would lead us from room to room, stopping at each table or drawer or whatever looked interesting. I supposed it was so important to him because he had never crawled or crept around. He had been stuck in one place unless I carried him. He still couldn't get to sitting or standing from the prone position without help. But he had normal curiosity and normal energy, and now that he had discovered how to put one foot in front of the other, he intended to make up for lost time. He seemed happier, less fussy, since he had found this new freedom. Fortunately, his right leg didn't appear to hinder him. It toed out and dragged a little, and he got off it quickly, but that was minor. At least he would walk, and soon too.

Since Jamie was progressing reasonably well, Alden and I decided that it was time to have a second child. In February, we learned that another little Bratt would be born in October.

On the occasion of Jamie's one-year check-up, I angrily scolded my pediatrician for concealing facts from me or for not recognizing the facts himself, and informed him that this was our last visit to him. He did not defend himself. It was as though he was glad I had finally discovered the whole truth and he was thankful it hadn't been he who'd had to tell me. He suggested that I stop in at a nearby rehabilitation clinic to see if they might have a program for infants. I had never thought to go there. For me, a rehabilitation center was only for people who needed therapy after a sports injury or a car accident.

I visited the center on the way home and signed Jamie up to come in twice a week. Wednesday afternoons he was to be in a one-hour group session of mothers and babies with varying disabilities. Friday mornings he was to be seen individually for half an hour by a physical therapist. I felt satisfied that in addition to the home exercises we'd been shown how to do in Boston, we were finally doing something concrete for Jamie.

After only a few visits to the rehabilitation clinic, Jamie learned to get into the sitting position by himself. Soon he could also pull himself to a standing position. At 14 months, Jamie walked alone. At 16 months, he said his first two words, "Hi" and "a-boo." I was disappointed that he didn't say "Mama," but I imagined that he would learn to call me very quickly once the new baby arrived.

Meanwhile, my pregnancy was going well. Surprisingly, I was not constantly worried about the health of this child, as I might well have been considering the problems we were now dealing with as a reult of my last delivery. On Saturday, October 11, 1975, I woke up at 5:00 A.M. with labor pains. I had been scheduled to enter the hospital two days later for a repeat Caesarean delivery. I was relieved because I had feared surgery before labor might inadvertently deliver a pemature infant. At 8:15 A.M, Jennifer Susan Bratt was born: a not-so-delicate nine pounds ten ounces. Only five days after the surgery, we took Jennifer home. As I held both my children, and Alden held me, I felt there was nothing wrong in my world.

Jamie and Alden both limped. Some people suspected that the son had merely inherited whatever the father had. In truth, Alden limped from the pain and stiffness of osteoarthritis in his right hip, while Jamie limped from lack of control, diminished feeling, spasticity, and from a difference in the length of the two legs, the affected leg being about two centimeters shorter. It was perhaps good for Jamie's developing ego that his father also limped. He was spared feeling different too soon.

At our third six-month evaluation in Boston, in April 1976, just after Jamie's second birthday, the orthopedist thought that Jamie should wear a cast on his right leg at night to keep that leg straight, and a brace during the day to help him put his foot down flat. New ones would be made for him periodically as he grew. We were enthusiastically in favor of any device that might help him. Now we were really doing something tangible. We were not promised that these things would make Jamie walk completely normally, but we knew they couldn't hurt him. After a couple of sessions of measuring, molding, and fitting, we came home with the first cast and the first brace.

The brace required no adjustment period whatsoever. It was a simple piece of L-shaped plastic that fit inside his shoe, went up to the middle of his calf and fastened around the front of his leg with a velcro fastener. After I cut the top of his shoe to relieve the pressure caused by the extra space the brace took up, he wore it without complaining.

Was it our imagination, or did he really walk better immediately? Even he was pleased with it, and made a point of showing it to everyone. The only disadvantage of the brace was that he couldn't squat while wearing it.

Jamie's initial adjustment to the cast, on the other hand, was not nearly as easy. It was a heavy plaster cast that went from his foot—only his toes peeked out—to the top of his thigh. It was split into two separate pieces down the full length of each side, so that the top half fit onto the bottom half. Five buckled straps held it together. I had to cut the right leg off of all his blanket sleepers as they were too bulky to fit inside the cast. The first time I put him to bed with that cumbersome cast on, he went right to sleep and stayed asleep all night. It wasn't his nature to question or protest.

Evidently he thought it was just intended to be a one-night endurance test, and he was willing to humor me that one night. When I strapped it on his leg the second night, however, he looked at me in disbelief, and then started to wail. For the next two weeks he woke up several times in the night. Soon Jamie accepted the cast as a necessary nuisance and stopped fussing.

There was a giant billboard right where we turned off U.S. Route 1 to go to our house. It pictured a child in steel braces and on crutches, and was a plea to support the March of Dimes. What agonized me were the giant words BIRTH DEFECTS ARE FOREVER. I had to see that every time I drove home. I didn't need a constant reminder of what was already gnawing at my soul. I could only try to help him with the cast, the brace, the exercises, and whatever else anyone dreamed up for him. But I could never make what he had go away.

3
On and Off Phenobarbitol

We had continued to go to the rehabilitation center through a second spring and summer. The rehab professionals opposed most of the advice we had received in Boston. Boston told us to passively exercise Jamie's limbs, the rehab staff encouraged functional use of his limbs. In Boston they told us Jamie should wear a cast and a brace, the rehab staff hinted these were not necessary. I hoped by following everyone's advice we'd gain something.

One aspect of Jamie's development that both the rehab center and Boston agreed on left me a little bewildered. Both centers had speech departments that had observed and tested Jamie. Both declared he had no problems with his oral musculature. Yet I knew this child could not suck, spit, lap, kiss, blow, chew, or swallow normally. He drooled continually. He only chewed on the left side. He was lousy at licking an ice cream cone. He turned his head to the left to bite into an apple or an ear of corn. Why wasn't I given some instruction in exercises to improve these basic functions? Wouldn't the same exercises improve speech production too?

Early that fall I figured out how to partially eliminate Jamie's drooling. Several times a day I let him chew a small piece of gum. That stimulated the swallow reflex so that he didn't drool while walking around. I was amazed that the speech departments in Boston and at the rehab had not recommended this simple solution.

Later that fall, when Jamie was two and a half years old, the rehab center opened a nursery school. I was skeptical and felt that they should give Jamie physical therapy, not an academic program.

His teacher under this new program thought that Jamie was having "staring spells" that could be attributed to petit mal seizures. It was true that Jamie had a certain air of spaciness or confusion about him at times. He paused, as if to let information sink in before acting. To me, he never seemed out of touch; I thought this a sign of some sort of learning disability we had been warned about. Jamie's teacher reported her suspicions to Boston and the pediatric neurologist there scheduled Jamie for an electroencephalogram.

The doctor explained the many brain wave irregularities, especially on the left side, saying brain-injured people had irregular brain waves. He said it would look the same whether Jamie was having seizures or not. The EEG now was to serve as a basis for comparison after starting medication: a daily dose of phenobarbital for six months.

Alden and I were hesitant. We were talking about a powerful drug when there had been no confirmed petit mal seizures. The doctor showed us a couple of the pills and said, "We think of them as nothing more than aspirin." We agreed to try. After all, what did we know? We were just parents.

For the first month on phenobarbital, Jamie was extremely drowsy. Several times his head slumped forward and he fell asleep at the dinner table. His walking was also more unsteady than usual. After one month, the drowsiness lessened and he went back to his usual degree of unsteadiness. But his daydream like spells continued.

That December, we enrolled Jamie in a regular nursery school two mornings a week and cut his attendance at the rehab center to one morning a week. We were dissatisfied with the idea of placing him with other disabled children in one classroom. One child needed to learn sign language, another needed to learn to get his head up off the floor, and another to learn to walk with crutches. Instead, each group of children in an age grouping received instruction in readiness skills and socialization: a typical preschool curriculum. We felt his academic, social, and creative needs could be better met in a setting where he would be interacting with children reasonably free of physical and mental handicaps. I mainstreamed him at two and half years, a year earlier than I had anticipated his attending nursery school, and long before mainstreaming was in vogue. He went willingly and happily. Soon he could count to ten and recognize such offbeat colors as pink and brown.

If Jamie seemed mildly confused and disorganized before taking phenobarbital, he now seemed more so all that winter. He was slow to answer a question, not because he didn't know the correct answer but rather because he apparently had trouble decoding the question. He was easily disoriented. He couldn't remember which way led to the front door in his own home. His ability to scan was limited: he would drop his crayon on the floor and it would be right at his feet and he did not see it. He couldn't locate sounds. When I hid a music box in the oven or under the couch, he clearly heard it but could never find it. We doubted his behavior was due to seizures.

A repeat EEG in the spring when Jamie was three revealed no change in his brain wave pattern. We decided, with the neurologist's consent, to stop the phenobarbital. We lessened his daily dose gradually, and by July 1977, nine months after his first dose, he was completely free of it. We noticed many changes in Jamie almost immediately. His communication skills increased dramatically—his vocabulary grew, his sentences were not so telegraphic, his questions were more intelligent, and he was good at relating the day's events to Daddy when he got home from work. He was full of mischief, more alert, and more observant. He was much steadier on the porch and cellar stairways, and he never fell asleep at the supper table any more.

More importantly, Jamie suddenly seemed to be developing some control of his right fingers! I first noticed it when he willingly wrapped his fingers around the safety bar of his outdoor swing. I hesitantly presented him with one-inch wooden cubes and an empty box. With great effort and much trial and error, he picked them up and dropped them in with his right hand! Next, I showed him some very large pegs that went in a large peg board. This was harder because releasing his grip at the right moment was the most difficult part. He was successful 25 percent of the time, and we were ecstatic! There was no way of determining how much of this progress was due to a developmental spurt and how much could be attributed to the fact that he was no longer drugged. Encouraged by his new progress, I became more diligent than ever in working with him. Things were going very well.

My best friend Susan Berry and Alden's best friend Dick Hobson, both from Massachusetts, visited most weekends. They had grown very close to our children. They were both single and childless. Perhaps our children fulfilled an emotional need to be nurturing. Dick got into the habit of rising at dawn, or earlier, with Jamie and Jennifer, while Alden and I slept late on Sunday mornings. He even changed Jennifer's soaking diaper and got both children juice and cereal. He was calm, soft-spoken, slow-moving, and he charmed the children. He was so much like the famous television character Mr. Rogers in both looks and mannerisms. Our other friends envied us, and wished they too had an Uncle Dick who came to visit every weekend.

Jamie was well into his second year of preschool, and his third year at the rehab. Though he was definitely more alert since we stopped the medication, he was still a somewhat "spacey" child. I worried how much was due to the original brain damage and how much was due to having taken the depressant phenobarbital during the time when his brain was growing and developing most rapidly.

Another worry gripped me. For the first time, Jamie, now almost four years old, realized that the other kids on the playground were more physically able than he. To make this difference worse, that winter the orthopedist in Boston had a hand splint made for Jamie. It was an awkward plastic contraption designed to hold his wrist and fingers up and opened, instead of down and closed. It took three hours to mold the splint to fit his hand, and Jamie was on the verge of tears the whole time.

Things were beginning to add up to him—the cast, the brace, the tests, the exercises, and now the splint. He was different and he knew it. People around him were always explaining to others why he couldn't do something or why he wore that brace. He listened to all this and I wondered what kind of a mental image of himself he was forming. I was scared. I knew feelings of inadequacy could destroy a person.

4

The Seizure

"Oh, my God! Berneen, come here quick!"

There was genuine panic in Alden's voice. I leaped out of bed and ran into Jamie's bedroom. What I saw made me gasp. The whole right side of Jamie's body was jerking repeatedly and intensely. He was unconscious and his eyes were rolled up and dilated. His right eyebrow raised with each jerk. The bed was soaked around his mouth. I knew Jamie was having a seizure.

My breath quickened, but I knew what to do. He was not thrashing about violently, so he was not in danger of injuring himself. I put a wash cloth between his clenching teeth to prevent him from biting his tongue. I made sure he was breathing regularly.

I sat down on the bed beside him, trying to be calm, and waited for the seizure to be over. I knew one generally lasted only a few minutes, and then the child just went to sleep as if nothing had happened. After fifteen minutes, there was no change. Seizures were supposed to be harmless, but what about the effects of a prolonged seizure? And how long had this been going on before we came into the bedroom? I called the hospital emergency room. The nurse said to bring him in immediately.

I was relieved to see Jamie's pupils contract in response to the bright April sunlight as we drove down the street. That was an encouraging sign that despite the frightening length of the seizure Jamie's brain was still responding to external stimuli.

The emergency room doctor seemed perplexed by Jamie's condition. He checked Jamie's reflexes and vital signs; temperature 100.2, pulse 140, respiration 40. I wanted to scream at him to make Jamie stop. Instead I was mute. I stared helplessly at Jamie and prayed. My outward calm was betrayed only when I was asked to sign a treatment permission—I couldn't read my own signature! The doctor paged a pediatrician who was in the hospital, and we were all awaiting his arrival.

I suddenly noticed that Jamie's left side was now jerking a little. The doctor noticed too and gave him a shot of Valium in the right arm. There was no effect. The pediatrician finally came and gave Jamie a shot of phenobarbital. Almost immediately Jamie calmed and slept.

The pediatrician admitted Jamie to the hospital for two days for observation and to do several tests. After a spinal tap, he fell asleep again from the large dose of phenobarbital and from the exhausting seizure that had lasted at least two hours, maybe more. I picked up the little lump from the crib and held him in my lap in a rocking chair until a nurse came in to wake him for X-rays. I talked and laughed with him for the first time that day and found his mind intact. I called Alden, who had returned home earlier with Jennifer, so he could be as relieved as I was. Alden came in at 4:00 p.m. and together we held Jamie, read to him, fed him supper, and rocked him to sleep. I spent the next day at the hospital while Alden went to work and Jennifer stayed with a sitter again.

All the tests on Jamie were negative. There was no other cause for the seizure other than brain injury at birth. The doctor told us that since there was no way to know if this seizure was an isolated event or if Jamie was destined to have one a week, one a day, or even many a day, he would have to go back on the dreaded phenobarbital. I sighed resignedly. Seizures themselves were not dangerous, but the fall that the victim sustained as he began the seizure was potentially dangerous.

I was consumed with guilt and fear. Had I been sleeping peacefully in one room while Jamie had been convulsing for hours in the next? The doctor assured me that the length of the seizure was unimportant, as long as Jamie was breathing the whole time. It seemed that the phenobarbitol was necessary this time.

All that second day Jamie was stumbly and his speech was slurred. These symptoms were of course caused by his system having to adjust again to phenobarbital. Back to a daily nap and an early bedtime and a depressed central nervous system.

Jamie's speech and locomotion were improved the next day and I took him home. As I turned off Route 1 to go onto our road, I stared in defeat at the giant billboard that was still there, screaming its message to me, BIRTH DEFECTS ARE FOREVER.

5
Sinking Into Depression

In the fall we discontinued Jamie's attendance at the rehab preschool, and just enrolled him in his regular nursery school three mornings a week. Meanwhile, we continued taking Jamie to the Boston hospital every three months during the winter. We had a box full of outgrown casts and braces in the attic. Jamie was doing fine in all areas as far as they were concerned.

But we were skeptical of the cast, brace, and splint prescribed in Boston. I checked Jamie's leg on the occasional nights he did not wear his cast to bed. It was always relaxed and not tightly bent. Did he really need that cast? With the brace in his shoe holding his foot at a ninety degree angle, he could not squat to play or go up and down stairs normally. The splint was awkward to wear and so far had not changed how he held his hand when not wearing it. He still couldn't use his hand for much and it frequently felt cold to the touch. Not only had Jamie's doctor in Boston hinted that we should consider surgery on Jamie's right hand, but he had also said that he would be watching the difference in the length of Jamie's legs. If it became too great, he would recommend surgery to close the "growth plate" in his left leg—his good leg. He would be a little short, but he would limp less. I was willing to cut Jamie's shoes and pajamas so that his cast and brace could be worn, but was I willing to let them cut into his perfectly good muscles and bones? How much trust should one have in a doctor?

Ever since Jamie resumed taking phenobarbital, we were ambivalent about it even though we had been thoroughly frightened by his seizure a year ago. Was it wrong to stop the medication? What if he did have another single isolated seizure? We compared the risk of possible harm from that single isolated seizure with the possible effects of being drugged for two years out of five when the human brain was growing most rapidly. I couldn't bear the thought that we might unwittingly be deliberately assaulting his vulnerable brain. How much did doctors really know? I hated putting those two little white pills next to Jamie's plate at breakfast and at supper.

Jamie would be five soon. My little boy was going to go to kindergarten in a few months. Or was he? Because of his physical disability, Jamie would not be able to do many things his classmates could do. He had difficulty with scissors and page-turning. He couldn't suck his milk up through a straw and couldn't blow his nose. He couldn't pump a swing or climb the jungle gym. He was tactilely defensive meaning he tightened and folded up and became a bundle of jagged elbows and knees when touched, especially when overstimulated. His vision, hearing, and speech were not perfect. He drooled (gum chewing would be taboo in school), wore a leg brace, and limped. Would he be an object of ridicule? And if all this wasn't enough to thwart his adjustment to kindergarten, he was possibly a seizure waiting to happen.

More importantly, Jamie was easily distracted, slow-moving, disoriented, and disorganized. Would he be able to find his way to the gym or the bathroom? I couldn't let him cross our street alone because he couldn't remember to look both ways and to listen. He frequently looked up into the trees or down a driveway. If I asked him to listen and tell me if it was safe to cross, he might say it was okay, when in reality there was a ten-wheel dump truck bearing down on us. He often stepped in front of a moving swing or vacuum cleaner or tricycle. Could I really let this child go off alone on a school bus?

BIRTH DEFECTS ARE FOREVER, the billboard taunted.

I was tired of driving to Boston. I was tired of the thirty-minute wait for the five-minute visit to the orthopedist, who wiggled Jamie's leg and watched him walk and then smiled and said Jamie was doing just great. Each cast required three trips to Boston. One to make the skeleton cast, one to pick up the finished product a week later, and one after three months to check that his leg had not grown too rapidly before the six-month period was up and it was time again for a new cast. Jamie was on his fourth cast now.

We felt we needed a closer orthopedist. I made an appointment with a doctor whose office was in the next town. He carefully questioned me and thoroughly examined Jamie. Then he made one more recommendation.

"One of the best things we can do for these people, Mrs. Bratt, is to teach them to use their pockets."

"What do you mean?"

"The afflicted hand is less conspicuous if it is out of sight in a pocket, and since he'll never be able to do anything with it anyway, that is a good place for it."

I was dumfounded and furious. Was this all the medical profession had to offer my son?

We were ripe for anything that might come along.

At a Christmas party a few months earlier we had met a smooth-talking chiropractor. He explained that most health problems were related to misalignment of the spine, and that proper care of the spine, along with good nutrition, was essential to good health. He admitted that he could not cure Alden's osteoarthritis in his right hip, but he was sure he could at least alleviate his pain and stiffness. As for Jamie, the chiropractor felt he might have more success with him as his whole problem might only be the result of pressure on a nerve in his spine. We jumped at the new hope. Though we had a negative preconception of chiropractic theory, we thought it worth the try. He was not pushing drugs or sorcery, so it couldn't hurt. In fact he said that Alden's daily consumption of Excedrin for pain was akin to putting perfume on manure. It was only covering up the problem. My grandfather had been a chiropractor and had been proud to hold license #1 in New Hampshire. My grandfather was also a hypnotist, but when I repressed that fact I found that I had a tiny pocket of respect left for chiropractors and was ready to get rid of the manure.

Alden and Jamie went for X-rays, and then spinal adjustments three times a week for two weeks at the total cost of 300 dollars. His office was too far away and his fees too steep, so, still believing in the theory, we switched to a closer chiropractor. The new man believed that the whole family should receive regular spinal adjustments because the purpose was not just treatment but prevention as well. So Jennifer and I went along as well. His policy for payment was to slip what you thought the visit was worth into a box with a slot in the top as you left. Alden faithfully put in ten dollars each time. We went for many weeks at the total cost of another 300 dollars. We joked that the lightening of Alden's wallet, which he carried in his right hip pocket, should lessen his limp.

But one day in mid-March, when I observed our chiropractor's nice Bahama tan, which he had been able to afford by using everyone's untaxable "donations", and when I noticed that Alden and Jamie were still limping out of the office, and limping all the way to the bank to make another withdrawal from our dwindling savings account, I decided enough was enough. Nobody felt any better and we were wasting our time and money.

Where could we turn now? What was left?

Faith healing. We had heard that a lot of people went to the jungles of the Philippines to see faith healers. They supposedly removed growths from people in operations that involved no cutting and no healing. Alden had a friend at the shipyard who had cancer of the lymph glands in his neck. He went to the Philippines in a last ditch effort to live. He came back cured. The lumps on his neck were gone and his doctors were amazed. While he was there, the faith healers had also straightened his teeth and cured his cataracts. He had movies that he had taken on the "doctors" pulling out malignancies with their bare hands. I saw these movies and they were very convincing.

We didn't have the thousands of dollars required to travel across the Pacific Ocean, but Alden's friend had the names and addresses of the faith healers whom he had met and would be willing to pray for a cure if they received a letter of explanation, a picture of the afflicted individual, and some money. Another friend of Alden's wrote for his mother, who had Parkinson's disease, and she went into remission. We quickly sent ten dollars to each of the three healers and waited.

Some time later, Alden's friend with the lymph cancer returned to the Philippines and caught one of the "healers" palming chicken innards — not patients' malignancies magically removed. He came home a desolate man and died a few weeks later. We eventually got our three canceled checks back — all endorsed only with and "X." What sort of jungle pleasures had they spent our 30 dollars on?

A deep feeling of hopelessness was growing within me.

6
The Crash of '79

I remember the night, shortly after Jamie's fifth birthday, that things finally fell apart for us.

Supper was in the oven waiting, and it couldn't wait much longer. Why wasn't he home yet? He said to expect him at seven and it was after eight. Alden frequently traveled for the government, and for years there had been occasional evening meetings—like when he had been president of the country club or when he had taught a boating safety course for the Power Squadron. So supper and I were used to waiting.

Jamie and Jennifer had been promised a good night kiss from Daddy, but had fallen asleep just before eight. A busy day of sliding on unexpected spring snow had quickly exhausted them.

That must be it—the snowstorm! Poor driving conditions were undoubtedly delaying Alden's return home. His flight from Washington had been due at five, and from there he would have gotten into his car that he had parked there two days earlier and driven the last two hours of his journey to Maine. I went to the phone in our bedroom. I first had to check flight arrivals, then traffic accidents. When I picked up the receiver, I heard only silence. The phone must have been knocked off the hook downstairs, who knows how many hours ago!

Now my anxiety was doubled. Maybe the state police had been trying to call me about a terrible accident and couldn't get through. I always panicked and thought the worst. I remembered that only a few months ago Alden had been flying to San Diego on the very same afternoon that the biggest air disaster in United States history took place at San Diego Airport. I had been petrified when I had heard the news on the radio. I had cried silently with relief when Alden finally called me and told me his flight had come in about an hour after the ill-fated one, and that he had seen the smoke from the wreck as his plane landed.

Now, no sooner had I replaced both receivers when the phone began to ring.

"Hello?" Was it Alden or the police my voice asked.

"Hi, Sugerplum. I've been trying to reach you for an hour."

"The phone was off the hook. Oh, I'm so glad everything is okay."

"Well, the plane was late getting in, and the traffic out of Boston was jammed up. I tried to call you from the airport and later from a gas station on Route 1 so you wouldn't worry. I'm at the Hampton Toll Plaza, so I should make it in about half an hour."

"Have you eaten?"

"No, not since lunch."

"Good I've got beef burgundy and baked potatoes in the oven."

"One of my favorites. What about some wine?"

"Yes. That's part of the plan."

"And how are my little offspring?"

"Sleeping now. Jamie couldn't believe snow in April."

"Neither can I. Well, I'll see you in a few minutes. Bye. Love you."

"I'll be waiting. Bye. Love you."

I watched for slowing headlights out of the living room window, and when I saw them I ran to the front door. As we embraced, Alden said, "You certainly did a wonderful job of shoveling, Mrs. Bratt."

"I had a little help from a five-year-old and a three-and-a-half-year-old. Come. Let's eat."

"I will in a minute. I want to check the kids."

He went down the hall and I went to the kitchen. I put the salad, potatoes, and beef burgundy—which looked like it had survived the extra hour and half of cooking—on the table.

"Alden, come on."

I lit the candles and took a bottle of Pink Catawba out of the refrigerator. I was starved, so I sat down and helped myself to the salad. I hadn't eaten since I had finished off the kid's supper four hours ago.

"Alden, it's after nine. I'm eating."

There was no answer. I got up to go drag him to the table. He wasn't in Jennifer's room. She was in her usual position—covers kicked off, knees tucked under her, bottom up in the air. I peeked into Jamie's room. In the dim light going into his room from the hall light I had switched on, I could see Alden kneeling on the floor beside Jamie's bed. His head and arms were on the bed and he was crying.

I froze. I didn't know why he was doing this, and yet at the same time I did know. I just didn't want to handle it now. I knelt beside my husband and put my arms around him. I wanted to comfort him and yet remain dissociated from the scene. I did not want to cry too.

"I love him so much. I just can't stand to think of all the things he can't do now and all the things he won't be able to do in the future. He looks so beautiful and innocent lying here."

I couldn't say anything. I was biting my lip too hard. Alden's sobs were not subsiding.

"Sometimes I think why him or why us. But it's not that. We can't change that. I just want him to be happy in spite of everything. He is now, but will he be later?"

I looked at Jamie. Thank God he was a sound sleeper. In contrast to his sister, he slept on his back, straight out, and seldom moved. How could he in that cast?

Suddenly, the reality of the situation swept over me. This was my son, my husband, and my problem. My mind raced. I saw a giant billboard that said, BIRTH DEFECTS ARE FOREVER, and under that slogan were pictures from Jamie's life. I saw his traumatic birth, which in fact I had missed. I saw him in a class with severely handicapped children. I saw him dozing in school and at the supper table. I saw him being operated on to rearrange good muscles. I saw him standing dejectedly apart from his peers. I saw him in a roomful of graduated casts. I saw him with his hand in his pocket.

I cried and the beef burgundy got cold.

PART II

ON THE PROGRAM

7
Renewed Hope

In the short history of enlightened treatment for the brain injured, in addition to the name of Dr. Temple Fay and others, the biographies of Dr. Glenn Doman and Dr. Carl Delacato will also need to be recorded some day.

Wolf, 1968, p. 227

Oh, how the warmth and relaxation of summer could sooth, and even temporarily erase, one's worries and heartaches. In July we celebrated some very joyous news: I was pregnant! Though I felt lousy, I couldn't have been happier. And it was made even more perfect by the fact that the baby was due February 20, which was my father's birthday and Susan's birthday as well!

Alden and I felt a renewed sense of hope that summer, not only because of the new life within me, but also because of a discovery that would temporarily but profoundly alter our life style and our judgment. The discovery was a book called *What to Do About Your Brain Injured Child*, by Glenn Doman.

Glenn Doman was a physical therapist who very early in his career had become discouraged with the lack of improvement shown by victims of stroke when receiving traditional therapies. Why was he exercising uninjured muscles in the arms or legs, or encasing them in braces or crutches, when the injury was in fact in the brain, he asked himself. After many years of around-the-world research which put him and his associates in contact with tribal cultures as well as sophisticated societies, he developed a theory of brain development that was unique.

Glenn Doman recognized that all information enters the brain through five sensory pathways—olfactory, gustatory, visual, auditory, and tactile, the latter three being the most significant input pathways for humans. A person's ability or disability is measured by his output in the areas of mobility, language, and manual competence. This output by the brain is dependent on the quantity of input via the sensory pathways. The greater the input, the greater the output. The rate of brain growth is not predetermined. In fact, said Doman, as brain growth could be slowed down by an injury (since the brain would then presumably receive less sensory input), so brain growth could be accelerated by a program of excessive sensory stimulation—particularly of the visual, auditory, and tactile pathways, and by frequent motor opportunity, particularly in mobility, language, and manual competence. In other words, if a child or an adult became brain injured at some point (whether before birth, during birth, or at any age after birth), the cure was simply a matter of increasing the sensory input to the unused brain cells, or programming, as one programs a computer. We all have millions of these unused cells, and they could be programmed at an accelerated rate to take over the functions of the brain cells that were damaged.

After much trial and error of various innovative ideas, Doman decided that the most effective sensory programming should consist of crawling on the tummy, creeping on all fours, brachiating (swinging from rung to rung on an overhead ladder), running, patterning (prescribed movements by three to five adults of the child's limbs while he lies on a padded table), masking (fitting a plastic bag over the child's nose and mouth for short periods so that he rebreathes his own carbon dioxide), and the use of flashcards (cards with words or pictures designed to teach the child to read and to increase his intelligence). Unnecessary drugs should be eliminated, and a strict vitamin and dietary regimen should be followed. All the background research and the resulting techniques were logically and convincingly explained in Doman's book. It would be further explained and demonstrated by Mr. Doman and his staff if a child became enrolled at his Institutes for the Achievement of Human Potential in Philadelphia, after which the parents would go home and spend eight to ten or even 12 hours a day working with their child and preparing materials for him. They would go back for periodic reevaluation and reprogramming.

The definitely strange methods of the program, the fact that it was carried out by parents and not trained therapists, and the fact that the program consumed so many hours a day were the three reasons that the Institutes' program was controversial and not well received by the medical profession. We found that out by inquiring about the Institutes at the rehab clinic and at the Boston hospital. But what had the conventional medical approach or traditional therapies done for Jamie or the rest of us? I couldn't think of a single achievement of Jamie's that I was willing to attribute to anyone's work but our own. If the Institutes' methods were somewhat bizarre and the hours strenuous, at least nothing about the program could hurt Jamie, even if it never helped him. The book gave examples of many cases where dramatic improvements had taken place while a child was on the program, and hinted that total cure was possible.

Total cure! Maybe birth defects were not forever as the billboard had told me and the world. Maybe cosmetic operations to rearrange good muscles were not advisable. Could total cure really be possible for Jamie? Alden and I debated that point, and whether or not to apply for acceptance to the Institutes, all summer.

Meanwhile, the book gave me the strength to do something I had long wanted to do. I abruptly discontinued Jamie's exercises and his use of the cast, brace, and splint. I simply put them away one day early in August, and didn't tell anyone except Alden, Susan, and Dick. At Jamie's next appointment in Boston early in September, the orthopedist gave his usual assessment. "Doing fine, Mrs. Bratt. Great flexibility and range of motion. Great job!"

It was not my intention to confront the man with the fact that all of Jamie's devices were now sitting in the attic as mementos. In fact, I let this doctor go ahead that day and make a new cast for Jamie's right leg. As I left that afternoon, I knew we wouldn't be back and that Jamie would never wear that cast. Instead of going to Boston again to pick up the finished cast when the office called two weeks later, I asked that it be mailed to me. The long box arrived by UPS a few days later, and went directly to the attic unopened.

The day after I returned from Boston feeling so smug and confident, I called the Institutes. I was too impatient to write. I was told to send them a complete history and description of Jamie to help them make a preliminary decision as to whether Jamie was brain injured (having a normal brain at conception), brain deficient (never having had a normal brain), or psychotic (having a normal brain but being emotionally disturbed). If they ruled out the latter two categories (which their program could not help), then they would send us the date of Jamie's first appointment, which would unfortunately be at least a year away, unless a cancellation occurred. The fee for the initial week-long evaluation and program would be $450 plus hotel accommodations. They would provide daily lunch and dinner for the three of us.

I spent several days composing the required detailed account of Jamie's life. I ended the letter with, "He is now becoming more aware of his inabilities and limitations. We fear frustration and ego damage to this happy child. The need to help him becomes more urgent each day." As I put the red flag up on my rural mailbox, I prayed for a speedy response and an early opening on the waiting list.

8
Good News!

Symptomatic treatment of such patients must be discarded at this point in medical history, not alone because it is unmedical, unscientific and irrational but, more pertinently and factually, because it has not succeeded in producing practical results.

LeWinn, et al., 1966, p. 72

Jamie came into our room at 5:30 a.m., completely dressed and the most bright-eyed I had ever seen him. It was his first day of kindergarten! He had on the new plaid pants and navy blue jersey that I had laid out the night before. I often marveled at his self-taught ability to dress himself.

As I cooked his scrambled eggs and cheese, Jamie babbled incessantly about the "big yellow bus" that would soon come for him. At 7:30 a.m. we all went outside. It was sunny, but the temperature reminded us that summer was over. Jennifer came out in her pink fuzzies, and Alden delayed his usual 7:15 departure for work. When the big yellow bus came into sight through the green trees, and the red blinking lights came on as it slowed in front of our house, tears suddenly came rolling down my cheeks. I hid behind my movie camera and captured Jamieson eagerly waiting for the bus to come to a full stop, and then excitedly climbing aboard without ever looking back.

At the end of the week, Mrs. Tarbell reported that Jamie had made a good initial adjustment to the morning routine and that he had made some friends. There was a special aide in the classroom, whom we had requested during the summer, to help him overcome his distractibility so that he could follow directions and complete his tasks.

In the last week of September, I had amniocentesis at a clinic in Boston. Even though this test was not routinely done on pregnant women until the age of 35, when the risk of producing a damaged fetus was greatly increased, I felt I had several valid reasons for insisting that my obstetrician arrange it. I was 32 years old, and the probability of producing a child with Down Syndrome at that age was about 1 in 800, as compared to 1 in 365 at the age of 35. Who should draw the line between what was acceptable risk and what was not? I already had a child with a mild disability (though not genetic) who required extra time every day, and who, when we went on the

Institutes' program, would require an extreme amount of extra time every day. I did not have the time or the emotional strength to devote to an even more seriously disabled child. I didn't want to be faced with the decision to terminate the pregnancy or not, but if the odds turned out not to be in my favor, and if I did decide to carry the baby anyway, at least I would have time to prepare myself.

The results of the test would not be available for several weeks. We asked also to be informed of the sex of the child. It was a bonus item that they could determine when they examined the baby's cells in the amniotic fluid. I already had a strong feeling what the sex of the child was, but I couldn't stand the fact that it would be written somewhere and that someone would know. I had to know too.

Five days later, I felt our baby move for the first time. That was when real attachment began for me. I prayed every time the phone rang that I wouldn't hear heartbreaking news from the laboratory in Boston.

While we waited to hear, Jennifer began attending nursery school two mornings a week. She had long been jealous of Jamie's going to school. She was thrilled to finally be part of the game. I was proud of her maturity and capability, but feared that she, too, was suddenly growing up too fast.

I have always remembered Jennifer's fourth birthday in October for a special reason. It was that morning, while I was making the cake, that I got the call from the clinic in Boston informing me that my baby was genetically sound! Relief and joy flooded through me as I sat on the edge of the bed. She asked me if I still wanted to know the sex of the child. I said yes, and she told me that I was carrying a male child. After I hung up the phone, I floated on my waterbed for a few minutes in a sort of trance. I felt like I had just been introduced to someone new, someone very special. It was no longer just "the baby" that was kicking inside me. It was my son, Benjiman Bernard Bratt.

There was more good news next month. We were accepted by the Institutes for the Achievement of Human Potential! It was now November 1979, and our first week-long evaluation and programming was scheduled for November 1980, a whole year away! What were we to do in the meantime? We were elated and frustrated at the same time.

If applying to the Institutes meant we believed in their philosophy, and if paying the required deposit meant we were committed to keeping our appointment to learn more about their philosophy, then didn't it follow that we should no longer continue with any measures contrary to their philosophy? This logic (along with the proven fact that Jamieson was doing as well without his cast and brace and exercises as he had with them) convinced us to eliminate the last remaining treatment that Jamie was currently enduring: the mind-dulling phenobarbital.

I called our neurologist in Boston and explained my doubts about phenobarbitol, and for the second time got his permission for gradual discontinuation. Hallelujah! Jamie could be just Jamie now, and subject to no outside influences or therapies.

After he had been in school for a few months, it was quite clear that he was not doing well. Mrs. Tarbell strongly recommended that he repeat kindergarten. Jamie's social and academic problems were more noticeable and significant than was his physical disability. Socially, he was immature and inappropriately silly, and academically, Jamie was unable to print or even recognize most letters and numbers, and had no ability to read simple words. The school had tested him. He was intellectually sound, but he apparently was going to have difficulty learning in the usual classroom situation. Could the Institutes fix that too, I wondered. We were confused, so we shelved the final decision about keeping him in kindergarten until June.

Meanwhile, we felt that valuable time was being wasted. Every day that Jamie was not improving in some way meant that he was falling further and further behind his peers. He was stagnating while we waited to become part of the Institutes' program. We had boldly abandoned his cast, his brace, his splint, his exercises, his phenobarbitol, and his evaluations at one of the finest medical centers of the world. He was now ours to mold, and we began to formulate a plan.

9
Getting Ready

Merely maintaining the individual at the level of his capability without exposing him to the environmental stimulation which will cause him to achieve his full potential is just another aspect of deprivation.

LeWinn, et al., 1966, p. 69

Through one of Susan's sisters, we heard of a family that had been on the Institutes' program and had successfully cured their child. We contacted them and met them in their home in January. The mother was exuberant and bubbly, and sincere in her belief that Glenn Doman could cure any child, including children with Down Syndrome. According to her, their five-year old son had a scissors gait, could not hear or speak well, had dozens of seizures a day, and had experienced some visual problems. In less than a year on the program he had been made completely well and was able to enter public school. He was now seizure-free, an A student, and played on the softball team. We watched him run and climb, we talked to him, and we listened to him read. Although we had no way of being sure just exactly what he was like before, he certainly seemed normal now. Could her story really be true?

She showed us her reading cards, hundreds of them, the plastic masks, which looked like modified sandwich bags with a piece of elastic that tied behind the head, the high, padded patterning table, and the 12-foot brachiating ladder, both built by her husband following the Institutes' diagrams, and both still set up in their living room though they no longer used them. She recommended that we begin subscribing to Ranger Rick, a children's magazine full of animal facts and photographs, and to Safari Cards, a monthly packet of 30 or so cards, also containing vivid animal photographs and interesting facts. We would eventually need them for the intelligence part of the program. She described what a typical day was like on such a strenuous program. Her enthusiasm was contagious and we felt reassured that we had made the right decision by applying to the Institutes.

She also shared another stunning bit of information. I mentioned just by chance that one of Jennifer's eyes was crossed and that I gave her daily eye drops. She assured me that the program could cure crossed eyes! Their own younger, healthy son had crossed eyes and the Institutes had told them to have him crawl, creep, and brachiate along with the older son. Sure enough, the condition had disappeared in only a few weeks. Was this all for real, Alden and I asked each other with our eyes. Was there nothing a little crawling and creeping and brachiating couldn't straighten out?

We had been toying with an idea for several weeks. We made the final decision on it that day. We could not wait until November. We would start the program now, on our own.

Our new friends taught us how to pattern Jamie, and generously gave us their table for as long as we would need it. While Alden took precise measurements of the ladder and made a list of tools and building materials he would need to buy, I wrote down what their son's first program had been: 80 one-minute maskings a day, seven minutes apart; six five-minute patternings, done by three people, spaced throughout the day; one hour of crawling; one hour of creeping; one hour of hanging on the rungs of the ladder; and one hour of reading.

That added up to six hours a day! No parent I knew ever spent that much time working closely with one child. I rarely had the time for the few minutes his old exercises required. Jamie got home from kindergarten at 11:00 a.m., so there were enough hours left in the day for the new program. But was there enough dedication in our souls? What would I have to give up? Time with Jennifer? Reading a good book? Cooking fancy meals? Shopping? Daydreaming?

Though six hours seemed like a lot of time, the mother of the cured boy said that after only a month on the program they had seen such huge improvements that they had actually doubled the time they spent doing the program! Such results were at least worth crossing cooking, shopping, and daydreaming off my list. We left their house with the patterning table tied to the roof of Alden's car, a bagful of plastic masks, resolved minds, and a very apprehensive son.

In one month Benjiman would be born. I was too exhausted and sickly to do anything with Jamie now. Most nights I went to bed before Jamie and Jennifer did, and they came in to kiss me goodnight. We needed that month to get organized anyway. The preparations required just to initiate the program were almost as staggering as the program itself.

The first thing we did was to buy a chin-up bar for the doorway to Jamie's room. It would have to do until the ladder was built. It was not easily removed, so any adults who entered had to duck. I had Jamie try to hang from it with both hands as many times as possible every day. He was exasperated when acrobatic Jennifer did somersaults through her arms on it and hung by her knees. He often forbade her to even use it.

We wanted to record Jamie's efforts on the program from the very beginning, and so I got my camera out to take a picture of his first attempt to hang. I wrapped the fingers of his right hand around the metal bar and stepped quickly back to snap the shutter. He could not even hang on for that short a time. I got back a picture of him dangling in his doorway by one hand. We had a long road ahead of us.

I wrote a quick note to the Institutes, informing them we had met one of their successes and that we wanted to start a program on our own. I wanted their blessing and assurance that we wouldn't be doing anything detrimental to Jamie. I received a prompt reply stating that anything we felt confident doing was okay with them.

Having received this official sanction, we plunged into the task of converting the small storage room off the TV room downstairs into a therapy room. We were lucky to have that space. We'd seen one family and heard of others who had ladders and patterning tables in their living rooms and kitchens. Our therapy room-to-be contained my sewing machine, a large built-in desk that jutted out into the room, and several large toys. All of these things had to go. Alden spent a whole weekend ripping out the built-in desk, and then repairing the wall it had been attached to. The following weekend he built the ladder. It had to be hand made because the dowels needed to be of a certain size and a certain distance apart, and because its height off the floor had to be adjustable.

Alden and Dick moved in the heavy patterning table. The small therapy room was just barely wide enough to accommodate both the ladder and the table. Then I handed Dick and Alden a roll of white adhesive tape and had them lay down one path that went around the table and one path that crisscrossed in a figure eight under the table. That was to give Jamie a visual reference while creeping and crawling. Next, Alden put up the large round clock, the type that is in every classroom in the country. I had bought that and a bell timer because the creeping, crawling, reading, and hanging was to be done in alternating timed segments, and not all of one thing for the full hour at once. Who could, or would want to, crawl for an hour straight? Finally, I taped to the wall a complicated sequencing chart that I had created showing what Jamie was to do for each one-minute and five-minute period for six hours, until all the quotas were met. There was space after each listed task to check it off when it was accomplished. It suddenly occurred to me, as I proudly explained it all to Dick and Alden, that in reality this program would take somewhat more than six hours to execute. I had not figured into my efficient and rigid schedule any time for transition from one activity to another, any time to go to the bathroom, any time to eat a snack, or any time for a hug.

Patterning required three pairs of hands to manipulate Jamie. On weekends, Susan or Dick or both would help us. During the weekdays, Alden didn't get home until 5:00, and it seemed logical to complete as much of the program as I could before that time. In order to accomplish the six five-minute patternings, I would need two helpers for about two hours every afternoon. Ten people in all for the week. I didn't know my neighbors very well, and my friendships in the area were only casual. I placed an ad in our small town newspaper that read, "Volunteers needed to help in home therapy program for disabled child." These were times of unemployment and inflation, and Alden thought I was crazy to expect anyone to come without being paid, no matter how noble the cause.

The newspaper came out about 3:00 p.m., and I sat expectantly by the phone at that time. No calls came that first day, but over the next several days, I received nine calls. Two were from people who said that they were interested but "had to think about it"; they never called back. Two were from people who just wanted to inquire and to wish us luck. One was from a woman who had done the program with her son fifteen years ago and asked to meet us but was not interested in becoming involved again. And four of the calls were from women who definitely wanted to help Jamie. It wasn't the ten that I needed, but it was a start. I arranged interviews with those four people. I wanted to meet with the people I would be letting into my home each week, and I wanted to inform each person more extensively about the program and show them the equipment and exactly what patterning was. Then they could decide for themselves if they really wanted to offer their time. Some of the women were fearful that the therapy would be strenuous, and were relieved when they saw how skinny Jamie was and that they would only be required to move an arm and a leg or his head, while the bulk of his weight rested on the table. I met them all in the few remaining days before Benjiman's birth, and each said she would be delighted to help.

Jeanne was a nurse, whom I had already met because our daughters went to the same nursery school. I hadn't been bold enough to ask for her help, but she had seen the ad and had recognized my telephone number. Etta had patterned for another family many years ago. Pattianne was hoping to be an occupational therapist and was interested in learning about alternative treatments. And finally, there was Cora Jo, who noticed a reproduction of my wedding invitation on the wall (giving my parents' names) and told me that she had graduated from the business college that my parents had owned. My father had solicited her as a student and my mother had taught her several courses. These four women were to be my helpers for the patterning sessions.

Cora Jo and Etta would come on Mondays from noon until two. Etta, sensing my shortage of volunteers, insisted on coming on Tuesdays at noon as well, with Jeanne. I had no one for Wednesdays. Pattianne could come on Thursdays and Fridays late in the afternoon when Alden was home from work to be the third set of hands. I was pleased that I had six out of seven days covered. Everything was set except for the starting date. I predicted that it would be some time early in March, and I told them I would call them sometime after the birth to let them know exactly when I felt well enough to begin.

I also met the mother who had done the program with her own son many years ago. He had cerebral palsy to a similar degree as Jamie, and was now in college. She moved and spoke slowly, with a mysterious sadness in her eyes. The program had helped her son, but hadn't cured him. She hinted that the stress of doing the program had contributed to her divorce from her husband. She listened silently to my enthusiasm and hopes. I had the distinct impression that this melancholy stranger was trying to warn me about something, but was restraining herself. She said goodbye, and I knew I would never see her again.

It was now nearing the end of February. Alden and I stood in the therapy room one evening after Jamieson and Jennifer were asleep. In our silence I knew Alden and I were thinking about the same questions. How could masking, creeping, crawling, and brachiating help cerebral palsy? Could any of that really have a permanent effect on the central nervous system? Such attention couldn't possibly hurt him, but how could it cure him? This skepticism had to remain unexpressed, hidden in the backs of our minds, so that it would not interfere with a total commitment to the new program. It was Jamie's last chance, and we intended to give it our all and to make judgments later. Alden looked at me, heavy with our third child, and then at the patterning table, on which rested the bell timer and our first issue of Ranger Rick, and then at the ladder. He said, very quietly, "I am awaiting the birth of one son, and the rebirth of another son."

10
Benjiman!

Every child born, at the instant of birth has a higher potential intelligence than Leonardo da Vinci ever used.

Doman, 1984, p. 24

The birthing policies of hospitals everywhere had become more humanized in the years since Jamieson and Jennifer had been born. Our hospital now offered rooming-in facilities for the mother and her newborn, specified visiting hours for siblings, any time visiting hours for father, and, most wonderful of all, fathers were now allowed in the operating room for Caesarean births. All that was required for that privilege was that we attend a one night class that included a movie and a discussion of Caesarean birth.

Benjiman's official due date was Friday, February 22. Repeat Caesareans were always scheduled one week in advance of the anticipated due date to assure that the mother did not go into labor. Labor could stress the old scar tissue into rupturing. If that happened, the baby would surely die, and the mother would need help very fast in order to survive. That meant the operation should be Friday the 15th. But it was very important to me to have this baby on the 20th, as it was Susan's and my father's birthday. My request to postpone the delivery to the desired day was granted, but I was told to take it easy and not to get very far from the hospital.

This was my golden opportunity to have the engraved birth announcements that I had always longed for. I had declined previously because there was too long a wait after the birth until the announcements were printed. But this time I already knew my baby's sex, and therefore his name, and I already knew the exact date that he would be born. The clerk in the Hallmark store was completely bewildered as I selected from her book a fancy vellum announcement, the one with the tiny footprint on the front, and dictated to her the name and date to be printed: Benjiman Bernard Bratt. Wednesday, February 20, 1980.

I received them a few days before the 20th. I eagerly addressed and stamped the envelopes. It was all I could do to resist mailing them!

I baffled another clerk, at the telegraph office. I arranged for two telegrams to be sent on Wednesday morning as soon as they got the go-ahead call from my husband. One was for my father and would read:

Happy Birthday to us,
Happy Birthday to us,
Happy Birthday dear Grandpa and me,
Happy Birthday to us!
Benjiman Bernard Bratt
Born Today

My father would be totally surprised because I had not informed him that we knew the sex or the date. Amniotic taps and due dates were beyond his realm of interest. He would be thrilled, I thought, with the unique birthday card. It was the type of thing he would do. He had once surprised my sister on Christmas by bringing a pony, with a big red ribbon around its neck, right into the living room where we were opening presents. And on my 16th birthday, before I even had my driver's license, there had been a little blue car sitting in the driveway when I had come home from school, with a sign on it that read, "Happy Birthday, Berneen. It's all yours!" Dad, whose given name was Bernard, would also be pleased to learn that his new grandson was named after him, as I had been named after him.

The second telegram was of course for Susan. She knew the name and the date, but still I knew that she would treasure the telegram.

Another advance at the hospital was that now they did an amniotic tap a few days before a scheduled Caesarean to check the LS ratio, which had to do with the maturity of the baby's lungs. The ratio had to be at least 2:1 to be sure that the child would not risk being born with hyaline membrane disease, a lung disease that kills many premature infants every year. This time it was not necessary to travel to Boston for the amniocentesis. Late in pregnancy it was more obvious where to stick the needle without hitting the baby, and my regular obstetrician did it. They had not done this test when I was expecting Jennifer. I was thankful that there was now a test that would make me confident that Benjiman was being born very close to his natural intended delivery date, instead of too early. There was no reason to doubt that the 20th wasn't right on target. Besides, I did not want to delay his arrival beyond the 20th. That triple birthday was very important to me.

I had the test on Friday, the 15th, and on Sunday, the 17th, my doctor telephoned me. My LS ratio was only 1 $\frac{1}{2}$:1! The 20th was canceled. Oh, Benjiman! I was so anxious to hold him in my arms and nestle him to my breast! It was a tremendous letdown and my depression showed. There would be no telegrams for anyone's scrapbook. And I had 75 birth announcements printed with "Wednesday, February 20, 1980." My extreme efficiency had finally exacted a toll. I tried to console myself with the indisputable fact that we were lucky not to be delivering a baby that was at risk.

The next few days dragged. On the 20th, I prepared a fancy birthday dinner for Susan and my father and tried to act cheerful. My next tap was scheduled for Tuesday, February 26. If the LS ratio was high enough, I could have my choice of delivery on Wednesday the 27th or the two suceeding days. I chose Wednesday the 27th because the announcements said "Wednesday" and I figured I could salvage them by gluing little scraps of paper cut from an extra announcement over the 0 in 20 and writing in a 7.

I went to the hospital early Tuesday morning for what I hoped would be my last amniotic tap. The doctor put in a rush request to the lab, whose report came at 3:30 p.m. The ratio was 5 $\frac{1}{2}$: 1—the highest the doctor had ever seen! Benjiman was ready! I checked into the hospital immediately.

At three minutes past 12 p.m., Wednesday, February 27, Benjiman Bernard Bratt was born. The nurse held him and I touched him. He had the same head of reddish-brown hair that Jamie had had when he was born. But I suspected that Benjiman, like his brother and sister, would be blonde before long. Too soon the nurse had to take him off to the nursery to be examined by the pediatrician. Word came back to the OR that Benjiman weighed just over seven pounds and ten ounces. Considering that I had gained 50 pounds again, as I had with Jennifer, I really expected Benjiman to be a little heftier.

Alden sat by my head throughout the operation, holding my hand. But instead of whispering in my ear as I imagined he would, his eyes were glued to the surgical site. He was totally absorbed by the skill and precision of the operating team. Later, he gave me a blow by blow description, including how they actually took my uterus right out of me and laid it on my abdomen to suture it.

Alden left for a few hours in the late afternoon to mail the announcements and to pick up our eldest two youngsters at a friend's. He had supper with them, left them again with a sitter, and returned to the hospital. He left around nine, and I settled down for a good night's sleep, at least until Benjiman's next feeding.

Alden wasn't to have it so easy. Shortly after he got home, both Jamie and Jennifer woke up crying. Jamie said he had an earache and Jennifer said that she itched all over. Alden gave Jamie gave some aspirin and then checked under Jennifer's pink fuzzies. She was covered with little red bumps. Not knowing what else to do, he gave her another bath; she'd had one earlier. There was still no improvement so he called our pediatrician. He said it sounded like hives and to give her a dose of Novahistine and a baking soda bath. So poor Jennifer had her third bath of the evening at 10 p.m.! It cured the itch. And in the morning Jamie had no earache. It had just been two individual expressions of nerves and anxiety over Mommy and the new baby!

The next day Jamie handed me a blue silk flower in a little vase. He and Jennifer peered at their brother through the glass, but could not touch him yet. Benjiman looked handsome with his long hair parted and slicked. He was already the doll of the nursery, just as Jamie had been six years earlier. Jamie and Jennifer were adorable, now dressed in their 3-D elephant sweaters that I had recently knit for them. It occurred to me that I should now make a third one. Suddenly I remembered that I probably wouldn't have time to do any knitting for a long while to come.

By Monday morning I was deemed fit to go home. I had planned a little birthday party for Benjiman to assure his welcome at home by his older brother and sister. I had already bought and wrapped a Barbie doll for Jennifer and a Superman puzzle for Jamie, both marked from Benjiman. And Jamie was giving Benjiman a squeeze toy and Jennifer was giving him a comb and brush set. The balloons and party hats and cake mix were all in the cupboard waiting to be used.

When my doctor visited me for the last time on his rounds that morning, he reminded me to take it easy for a few weeks and to be sure to get plenty of help at home. I enthusiastically nodded my agreement, but secretly I knew that I would have very little time to relax. What would he think if he had known about the physically and mentally demanding program we were about to embark on? In fact, I had even spent one afternoon at the hospital contacting all my patterners to inform them of our definite starting date.

We would begin the program on Monday, March 17, exactly two weeks from my hospital release.

11

April Instead of November

A precedent for reverting to the experiences of early infancy was established by Freud with reference to neuroses. If early psychological experiences affect the development of the psyche to the extent believed by most psychiatrists, it should come as no surprise that the early sensory experiences of infant behavior are of vital importance in developing the functional potentialities of the brain.

Thomas, 1969, p. vi

Considering the turmoil in our minds, Benjiman was the calmest and best natured of our three babies. Both Jamie and Jennifer had been on Donnatal for a short time to quiet their colicky stomachs. But Benjiman always went right back to sleep after being fed at night and seldom cried except to be fed or burped. Alden was as big a help as ever, getting up in the night, doing a very large share of housework and cooking, and always willing to change a diaper.

Benjiman put up with a lot of not-so-gentle loving from his big brother and sister, and never complained. I didn't put him back in his crib once he was up in the morning until nighttime. I let him catch naps when he could in his infant seat or swing during the daytime so that his long stretch of sound sleep would hopefully coincide with my long stretch of sound sleep, and I never insisted that Jamie and Jennifer be quiet because the baby was sleeping. I figured that the best way to minimize resentment was to make the baby adjust to napping through any level of noise around him rather than making those who were here first adjust to the new baby.

Jennifer was genuinely attentive to her baby brother. She always wanted to hold him or play with him or change his position for him. At only a few days old he actually cooed in response to her cooing as she laid on the floor beside him. It was an extremely touching exchange to eavesdrop on. Her movements were occasionally too quick or too jerky, but basically she was always careful with him and I felt that I could trust her around him.

Not so with Jamie. On Benji's second day home I came back into the living room from answering the telephone in the bedroom and found a blanket wrapped snugly around Benji's head! It would never even cross Jennifer's mind to do that. While Jamie would never intentionally hurt anyone, he needed to be watched because he didn't have a good comprehension of fragility or danger. Maybe that was why Benjiman was so quiet, he didn't want to draw any undue attention to himself!

Uncle Dick's paternal instinct was more in evidence than ever before. He was now much more experienced at such matters as maneuvering wiggling limbs into unyielding sleepers and transporting a baby in the useful football hold. Dick thought that the name Benjiman Bratt had a particularly poetic ring to it, so he composed a little nonsensical ditty that he often recited as he gazed fondly at Benjiman.

> Benjiman Bratt
> Grew awfully fat
> And he lost his hat
> Chasing Uncle Dick's cat—
> Now imagine that!
>
> But Benjiman Bratt grew awfully thin
> Before his hat was on again.
>
> Now sometimes he's mad
> And sometimes he's sad,
> But when he's glad—
> He wears a great big grin!

On Tuesday, March 11, I was bathing Benjiman in his little yellow tub on the bathroom counter when the telephone rang. Jamie ran for it and then came to tell me that it was my sister, Aunt Guilene in Philadelphia. I wrapped up Benji and headed happily for the phone.

Jamie had the city right, but the name wrong. It was the Institutes for the Achievement of Human Potential on the line. They had just received a cancellation for their next class, and since we were so eager, would we like to come for the week of April 21 instead of November?

The reality and enormity of our chosen path overwhelmed us as Alden and I discussed it that evening. We were scared, skeptical, nervous, elated, and hopeful all at once. We would still start on our own next Monday in order to get a feel for the program and thereafter be able to ask intelligent questions about it when we got to Philadelphia five weeks later.

As I tucked the children into bed, I prayed for Alden and myself to have the strength to do the program, for Jamie to have the strength to endure it, and for Jennifer and Benjiman not to feel too neglected by it.

12
Starting on Our Own

Environmental enrichment in the brain-injured human being must be much greater than that which produces maturational changes in the unaffected brain.
LeWinn, 1969, p. 208

On Sunday, March 16, we went through two hours of the program, using the sequence I had mapped out in the chart on the wall, to be sure there were no unforeseen glitches. Dick was here and he was the third for patterning. He stood at the head of the table, rhythmically turning Jamie's head from side to side. Alden and I stood on opposite sides of the table, Alden on Jamie's left and me on Jamie's right, which would be my permanent position for many months. As Jamie laid on his tummy, Alden and I each moved one arm and one leg in the prescribed manner that simulated crawling and creeping. We put Jamie through his other paces as well, and found no problems. We were all ready for the next day.

On Monday morning, March 17, when Jamie got off his bus at 11:00, I was at the door waiting for him with a mask in one hand and a timer in the other hand. I was supposed to put the mask on him for one minute, 80 times. Since there had to be seven minutes between maskings, it would take nearly 14 hours to do all 80. Jamie usually went to bed at 7:00, so in the eight hours remaining before 7:00, I could not possibly reach the quota. But in order to do as many as possible, I had to start right away. I slipped it over his nose and mouth, set the timer for one minute and bent down to unsnap his yellow slicker—it was pouring out—and to take his papers out of his hand, talking to him all the while as if there was nothing unusual happening.

At noon, Cora Jo and Etta arrived. I had masked Jamie seven times, fed Jamie and Jennifer lunch, nursed Benjiman again so that he would be content for two hours, and had put shorts and a short-sleeved shirt on Jamie because patterning was supposed to be done with bare arms and bare legs for maximum tactile stimulation. We all went downstairs to the therapy room.

The cold hit us in the face. We had two-zone heat and we seldom turned up the thermostat down there unless it was exceptionally cold when we wanted to use those rooms. Usually we just put on another sweater and heavier socks and built a roaring fire in the fireplace when we wanted to watch TV, instead of turning on the heat. But now I realized that with strangers in the house and with Jamie's skinny limbs exposed, it would be necessary to burn some oil. I felt embarrassed as I turned up the thermostat to 68 degrees, closed the fireplace damper, and then nestled Benjiman in a blanket on the floor in the TV room. Jennifer, appropriately dressed in green in honor of the date, plunked herself down next to Benjiman and remained reserved because of the newcomers and because of her uncertainty about what was about to happen. I too felt nervous.

I hoisted Jamie up onto the patterning table for his first official patterning. When I told him to please lie down on his tummy, he looked at me with resistance in his eyes. I repeated my command with my eyes and to my great relief he obeyed. I positioned Cora Jo on Jamie's left and Etta at his head, and went through the instructions for our synchronized movements again. When we were all ready, I set the timer for five minutes and we began. No one said a word, partly due to shyness and partly due to fear of jeopardizing our perfect rhythm and teamlike coordination. It was going so well until Jamie, who had only minutes earlier abandoned active resistance, decided to try passive resistance.

"Mom, it hurts to lay on my penis." His voice was somewhat muffled because of the way Etta was holding his jaws to turn his head alternately from one cheek to another, but we all heard what he said. Cora Jo and Etta were looking at me for a response. Should I obligingly offer him a cushion or should I denyingly point out that all men were able to sleep on their stomachs without such complaints? I chose the latter reply and won Jamie's silence for another minute. Then he tried again.

"Mom, even if righty gets better, I won't ever use it! So there!" There was a catch in his voice, as if he were about to cry. He knew that I could force him to do these physical things, but he was letting me know that I didn't have control over his mind as well. His defiance was understandable, and my heart went out to him. But we had made our decision and I could not give in or stop patterning. I muttered some palliative remark and stared pleadingly at the bell timer. Mercifully, it went off. Jamie sat up while I ushered Cora Jo and Etta into the TV room, telling them to make themselves at home and go upstairs for a cup of coffee until I called them into the therapy room again in ten minutes for the second patterning. Benjiman had fallen asleep and Jennifer was watching Sesame Street. I closed the door, on the pretense that Jamie would be distracted by Big Bird or Cookie Monster, but actually I felt a strong compulsion to proceed with our work unobserved since I wasn't entirely comfortable with what I was doing, and I wasn't sure how much discipline I would need to exert in order to accomplish the goals.

I put the plastic mask on Jamie's face for one minute, I helped him hang on the ladder for two minutes, and then I sat on the floor and chattered to him while he crept around and around the table, following the white tape, for five minutes. After I slipped the mask back on his face again and put him on the table, I checked off what we had done on my wall chart and opened the door to call in my volunteers for the second patterning.

The three of us took our positions around the table and waited for the minute to be up. The bell rang, and in one smooth motion I slid the mask up over Jamie's forehead with one hand, while with my other hand I pulled his two hands forward so he would land on his chest and be ready for patterning. Time was a very important factor and none could be wasted. I hastily reset the timer for five minutes and we immediately began to move Jamie's limbs and head. The three of us were more comfortable in our task this time, and we found that a little friendly conversation did not break our concentration. Jamie raised the same objections again. I squelched them with more vigor this time and he acquiesced.

Outside we could hear the wind howling and the rain beating. We were well into the five minutes when suddenly the lights and the TV flickered and then went out. It was nearly dark in the therapy room because there were no windows on the front side of the cellar, and only a little light reached us from the two windows in the next room. But we did not miss a beat in our patterning. We did not need to see; we only needed to feel and to hear. I was acutely aware of my own two arms extended away from the sides of my body as I held Jamie's right arm and right leg extended, and then, a moment later, of my two arms moving toward my waist as I bent Jamie's right wrist and right knee toward his waist. Jennifer came in and sat under the table near my feet. I jumped when the timer signaled that five minutes had elapsed.

I brought two candles into the therapy room, lit them, and Jamie and I continued in the shadows. Jamie did masking, hanging, and crawling this period. Crawling, which is hitching along on one's belly, is a much more strenuous activity than creeping—especially for one using only one side of his body. He made only five trips around the table in as many minutes, and he needed constant coercion to continue, in comparison to 20 easy trips around when he had been creeping.

Benjiman was still snoozing and Jennifer was building with the wooden blocks under the table when it was time for the third patterning of the day. Cora Jo and Etta put down their coffee and took their positions. We were laughing now about the dark room and the fact that nothing could stop us. Even Jamie seemed more jovial. This pattern was followed by more maskings, hanging, and creeping. Later, we did three more patternings, again followed by masking, hanging, and creeping or crawling, before it was two o'clock and time for my two volunteers to leave. Jamie and I spent the next three hours masking, hanging, creeping and crawling, with two short juice breaks and one long break while I nursed Benjiman and read to Jamie and Jennifer by candlelight.

The electricity came on again just in time to cook supper. As I chopped vegetables and shaped hamburgers, I related the day's events to Alden. We had not met all our quotas this first day, but we were too exhausted after supper to resume the program. Jamie's knees and elbows, unaccustomed to the constant abrasion of the carpet, were red and sore. I rubbed cream on these spots and tucked him in. I fed Benji again, and then tucked myself in and fell into a deep, dreamless sleep, until Benji's midnight feeding.

The rest of the week went smoothly, with Jeanne and Etta helping me on Tuesday, and Pattianne on Thursday and Friday. Because Pattianne was at our home from 4:30 to 6:30, we invited her to eat dinner with us both days, and she accepted. Alden fixed dinner between patternings, while I kept Jamie busy creeping and crawling and hanging.

Jamie could now keep his right hand on the rung beside his left hand for five to eight seconds. At the end of our first week on the program, he consistently kept his right palm down when creeping. Before the program he had had no control over that hand, and had always put the back of his hand down on the floor in an awkward, bent fashion. I captured this change on film for my records.

Jamie's sore elbows continued to be a problem when creeping or crawling, but with proper encouragement and distraction I persuaded him to endure it, promising him that his skin would soon toughen. I frequently told him stories, or made up games such as the drawbridge game where I sat in a chair with my feet up on the patterning table and he crept or crawled underneath. Sometimes I even crept or crawled with him, and we chased each other. I could already see that creativity and inventiveness were to be a vital part of the program.

Susan and Dick arrived for their weekend tour of duty. I was more organized by then and we were getting closer to achieving the quotas in the six hours that we worked with Jamie. I was the one who worked with Jamie because I was the best at coercing him. I only called on the others when it was time for patterning, or for a few minutes' relief while I fed Benji or gave Jennifer some attention. I took advantage of this luxury of being able to slip away, because I knew that on weekdays I would have to become adept at doing three things simultaneously—supervise Jamie's program, nurse Benji, and play with Jennifer.

The following Friday was Jamie's sixth birthday. It was his first out-of-the-house party. I didn't have the time or the energy for the preparation and clean-up that a party at home required. We faithfully did four hours of the program before leaving. Jamie loved pizza, so I planned a supper party at Papa Gino's at the mall. They let the birthday boy make his own small free pizza in the kitchen while his guests looked on enviously. I shot a memorable movie of Jamie tossing the dough and then spreading the tomato sauce and shredded cheese. His grin was the biggest I had seen since he started the program two weeks before. Alden came home from work early to accompany us. Having had no time to bake, I ordered a cake from a baker and carried it along with the ice cream.

At six o'clock, we left the mess behind and gathered up gifts and guests. We went home and did two more hours of creeping, crawling, masking, hanging, and reading with flash cards. Time spent was our criterion for quitting, rather than getting the specified amount done—and we always got less done in the allotted time than was scheduled to be accomplished, due to resistance or transitions or, in this instance, partying. Would Philadelphia reverse this flexibility? Would we have to meet quotas no matter how long it took? For the time being, fatigue took precedence over quotas.

The next day Susan and Dick came as usual. Dick had with him the best birthday present Jamie had ever gotten. Jamie loved boats and was fascinated with the two drawbridges nearby. Dick had made Jamie a working drawbridge, just the right size for his Matchbox cars and trucks to go over, and for his small boats to sail under. We were all impressed. We used it as an incentive all weekend. When Jamie finished a certain amount of work, he was allowed a few minutes to play with his new toy.

Doing the program all weekend after the excitement of his birthday party on Friday, and not being allowed to just play freely with his new toys, must have seemed cruel to Jamie. He was more balky than usual. Or maybe he realized that this creeping and crawling and hanging business was not just a temporary thing. Sunday afternoon, as he sat up on the table after the last patterning, he suddenly said to me through big tears, "I hate this! I wish I didn't have to do therapy! I wish Jennifer had to crawl and creep and wear the mask and do patterning!"

Jamie continued to make minor improvements. The countdown was two down and three to go for the Philadelphia trip. During week number three, he hung for 37 seconds one time. He even let go with his right hand and reached to the next rung and tried to hold on. That was the first step toward real brachiating. We seemed to have a new cause for celebrating almost every day. On April 4 he read his first book. It was a simple counting book, one dog, two chicks, and so on, up to ten, but he knew every word. He learned some of the number words while he was creeping and crawling around the patterning table. As he came around one end, there I was, sitting on the floor, nursing Benjiman and coloring with Jennifer and holding up the word card that told how many times he had been around the table. He looked at it without my even telling him to.

Jamie learned at least 20 other words as well. It had taken me time to realize that the reason Jamie was not reading sooner was that initially he was not even looking at the word cards—he was just obediently repeating the words after me while I was busy looking at each card! Once I started physically forcing him to look, which entailed a considerable battle, he had learned rapidly. I had started with silly words, to get his attention, but his silliness had been unbearable, so I had abandoned that tactic and stuck to common words.

Jamie was also inadvertently learning primary addition and subtraction. When I told him to crawl a certain number of times around the table, he told me how many he had left to do after completing each lap. I also saw him beginning to learn about telling time. Since everything was timed, he spent a great deal of time watching that big schoolroom clock on the wall. He counted the time for how many minutes he had to do something, and he took the mask off himself when one minute was up. He also knew when it was quitting time.

As the date neared, we made reservations at a hotel recommended by the Institutes and sent a deposit. We decided not to stay with my sister Guilene because she lived on the other side of Philadelphia and we didn't know how demanding our schedule would be. The itinerary we had received indicated that we would have meetings late into the evenings. Susan was accompanying us to Philadelphia. It was fortunate that our week-long appointment just happened to coincide with her spring vacation.

One aspect of the upcoming journey made me a little uncomfortable. We were not taking Jennifer. We would be terribly busy and she would be terribly bored. My friend Judi offered to take her for the week and we accepted. Of course I had to take Benjiman in order to feed him.

I planned to ask the proper person at the proper moment at the Institutes about Jennifer's eye that turned in. I hoped they could give me some advice about what aspects of the program might be of benefit to her without actually seeing her. We had just recently decided to stop putting drops in her eyes and to correct the strabismus with glasses instead. We were waiting for them to be made.

We had been told that this program put a strain on most marriages. In our case, so far, it had brought Alden and me closer together. We were just doing what had to be done. I did most of the therapy because I was better organized and because I had better control of Jamie. Alden did the laundry, vacuumed, swept, got supper, did the dishes, and worked at the shipyard eight hours a day. My two sons required all my time. There was not much time for my husband, my daughter, or for myself. The only time I had away from the program was while Jamie was at kindergarten from 7:30 until 11:00. I spent that time either with Jennifer, when she wasn't in nursery school, or doing errands. We guessed it would get worse before it got better. We expected a substantial increase in hours of therapy after our visit to Philadelphia.

There were two further signs of Alden's firm commitment to the program. Though I was driving Jennifer to nursery school in the morning after Jamie got on the bus, Alden was now picking her up and bringing her home during his lunch break, so that I would not lose any time with Jamie, who was home from kindergarten before she was out of nursery school. That was a tremendous help. But I knew my husband was truly serious about the importance of it all when he informed me that he had decided to give up playing golf for the summer! No Thursday night league and no Saturday morning foursome! That was a total sacrifice.

There would also be no more visits at my father's house or at Susan's or Dick's. We hadn't been anywhere since before Benjiman was born. We couldn't do therapy anywhere but at home. I cooked no more gourmet meals, the beds stayed unmade, and the kids seldom got a bath.

It was nearly time to pack for a trip that we believed would change all our lives temporarily, and Jamie's forever. Jamie's teacher, Dixie Tarbell, called me on Friday, two days before we were to leave. I was in the middle of our grueling, repetitious therapy and feeling a little down, overtired, skeptical, and scared of what the Institutes were going to ask of us and for what gain. So what if we made him the best creeper and crawler in town, I was mumbling to myself.

Mrs. Tarbell, who didn't know about the program we were doing, said she had noticed a remarkable improvement in Jamie in all areas in the past few weeks! His printing was legible, he could read simple words, he did his math papers correctly, and he frequently finished his work without assistance from the aide. He joined in with the other kids at recess instead of just standing there and staring. He climbed on the jungle gym and went on the seesaw and held on with two hands. I was thrilled at this report. I, too, had noticed some changes. He was now telling me more about his day when he came home. For example, that very morning he had known that it was his turn for show and tell. On his own, he had picked out a toy, put it in his bag, and taken it to school.

In order to go on, I had to believe that these changes were due to what we had been doing, that they were not merely developmental or coincidental. I believed it.

13
Bloody Monday and Terrible Tuesday

There is open to us today a means whereby, through environmental manipulation, neurological organization can be greatly improved both in the brain-injured individual and in the normal human organization.

LeWinn, 1969, p. 212

Sunday morning at 8:00 we were backing out of the garage, with Dick saying his last goodbyes through the car windows. Jennifer parted easily from us at Judi's, and we were soon traveling south to pick up Susan, and then we were officially on our way.

At 5:00 we passed through the enormous stone gate that was the entrance to the Institutes for the Achievement of Human Potential. Our appointment wasn't until 10:00 the next morning, but we couldn't wait. There were several stately ivy-covered stone mansions surrounded by beautifully kept grounds with flowering trees. Though we didn't see a soul, a sign warned "Speed Limit 5, Children Everywhere." We exited after a few minutes, feeling as though we had seen part of the promise ahead of time.

We checked into our hotel, and found it to be a very old building, probably not built as a hotel. Our room wasn't even as big as my kitchen. There was no pool, no lobby, no room service, no air conditioning, and no screens on the windows. Worst of all, we had only a double and a single bed in our room. I had made reservations for five and requested a crib. They had no other room available, so they moved in a rollaway bed and a playpen. Except for a small entryway, our room was now wall to wall beds. Alden and I literally had to climb over either Jamie's bed or Susan's to reach our double bed. When we went out to dinner we searched for an alternative but could find no vacancies. We consoled ourselves with the fact that this was not intended to be a luxury vacation and that we would be spending only a minimal amount of time in our room. What did it matter if some of us had to get dressed standing on our beds—the ceilings were plenty high.

We ate breakfast the next morning at a little cafe just a few doors down the street. We were to become regular customers of this plain but appealing establishment. The big round booth seemed less cramped than out hotel room. I nursed Benjiman while I ate my cheese omelet, and we listened to the morning news on a TV set behind the counter.

We parked at the Institutes and walked toward the impressive stone building where we had been instructed to gather with the other families. A pleasant lady handed us a three-ring notebook with a symbol of the Institutes on the cover and a list of the parents and children in our class inside, along with plenty of paper for note-taking. She led us into a dining room and told us to help ourselves to coffee.

We stole surreptitious glances at the dozen or so other families also drinking coffee and waiting. I looked at my blue plastic notebook. The symbol on the cover appealed to me. It was an adult hand opened palm upward with a small figure walking off it—as if to say that given a helping hand a child could progress. I looked inside at the list of names and addresses of the families with whom we were about to spend a week. I was astounded at the distances some had traveled. Of 29 families, only fifteen lived in the United States. There were two from Canada, one from Jamaica, one from Panama, one from Venezuela, two from Italy, one from Spain, one from Portugal, four from Japan, and one from the Republic of South Africa. I began to listen to the conversations at the other tables around us. They were not all in English. Could this place really offer so much hope that people could justify coming so far?

Alden and Susan were on their fourth cup of coffee at 11:00 when we heard our name called. A woman led us past the entryway through a lobby to a large paneled door. On the way she remarked to Jamie that Glenn Doman looked a bit like Santa Claus because he was overweight and had a white beard. I was delighted with the analogy because Santa always brought what you asked for.

Mr. Doman had an air of dignity and sincerity. He wore a vested suit and was one of those persons who always had a smile on his face. Jolly, I thought. His office was a bright sunporch, and I admired his large collection of stone and wood figures. They were all of human mothers and babes. Some were abstract and some were detailed. Some were obviously Western, while some were obviously African, Oriental, or Eskimo. He must have gathered them during his years of world-wide research.

He asked us some questions about Jamie and then he told us that he had much to teach us and that if we listened carefully we would learn more in this one week than we could in a whole semester at college. We would in fact receive a diploma. He winked as he confided to us that the reason his staff members constantly smiled was because they were so happy to be helping children. And, he said, the days ahead of us would be the happiest days of our lives, because we would know what our purpose in life was: "to save our kid."

Mr. Doman ended our brief visit by instructing our escort, who had remained present, to take us to meet our advocate. She led our little procession of five people, a diaper bag, a toy bag, and an empty stroller into a newer, angular building. Though we would be seen by many people during the week, our advocate, she explained, would be our main source of information and support. He was straight-faced, all business, and stricken with nasal allergies. He never smiled, avoided eye contact, and proceeded as if neither Jamieson nor Benjiman were present. For one and a half hours he asked me questions about Jamie's developmental history and laboriously wrote my answers down on a lengthy form. I had sent all of that information ahead of time—hadn't he read it?

Our advocate finally sent us to the dining room for lunch at 1:00 with the stern admonition to be back in the waiting room of his building by 1:30. We sat at a vacant table, eating quietly, wondering what was next.

What was next was a lot of waiting. The waiting room was bigger than a basketball court, with folding chairs along the walls and a big empty space in the middle. There were many other families waiting with us and each remained within its chosen space. There was no agenda and there was no way of knowing when or by whom we would next be seen. I was thankful for Jamie's toy bag.

At 2:30, a tall man led us to his office. For an hour he evaluated Jamie's functional abilities. He asked Jamie to read and write a little, and to creep, crawl, and run. He determined Jamie's eye dominance by asking him to peek through the keyhole, noting which eye Jamie used, his ear dominance by asking him to go listen at the wall to see if he could hear what they were saying in the next room and noting which ear he used, his leg dominance by asking him to kick a ball rolled toward him and noting which leg he used. He also tested Jamie's tactile sense by using a pin and a feather alternately on Jamie's feet and hands and then asking Jamie, who was not allowed to peek, which he felt. He also had Jamie reach into a cloth bag and try to identify objects by touch. The tall man marked his observations on a rainbow colored chart referred to as the "Developmental Profile."

Back in the waiting room again, I fed a hungry baby while Alden and Susan took Jamie out for a breath of air. There were brachiating ladders at several locations on the grounds and Alden wanted Jamie to practice hanging from one. There were also several patterning tables around the waiting room, but most mothers were using them as changing tables for their children because they, unlike us, did not know what other use they could have. The receptionist's office never had any idea when or by whom we were next due to be seen. So someone always had to stay in the waiting room to call the others when we were called. Between 4:00 and 6:00 that Monday we had three short, ten to fifteen-minute meetings with three different people who explained to us the different parts of the general profile used for all candidates.

The profile tested six areas of competence: visual, auditory, tactile, mobile, language, and manual. Under each area there were seven levels of competency, each level corresponding to a stage of brain development and an expected time frame for attainment. There was a total possible score of 42. All scores could be converted to a neurological age. Thus a child's extent and location of brain damage could be determined from this simple functional evaluation. Our last appointment before dinner was for a group picture for our file folder.

At 6:00 we were invited to supper, and told that at our last appointment, early in the evening, we would be informed of the staff's decision about Jamie's suitability for the program.

At 7:30 a woman beckoned us to follow her. Her spacious office was lit only by a small table lamp, where she sat studying Jamie's folder. We waited quietly in the shadows on a black leather couch. She looked up over her glasses and spoke her first words to us.

"I'm happy to tell you that your child is brain injured."

Perhaps we were supposed to jump for joy, but none of us moved. Of course what she meant was that since Jamie was judged not to be brain deficient or psychotic, he was therefore brain injured, and would benefit from their program. But she had an odd way of saying it.

She briefly explained to us, using a diagram of the brain with little X's, where and to what extent they felt Jamie was injured. This diagram and assessment were based entirely on the tall man's functional evaluation of Jamie.

She told us to return to the waiting room at 10:00 the next morning for another day of evaluations and explanations. Then Wednesday and Thursday would be spent in the auditorium listening to lectures by Glenn Doman and others. Children would be cared for in the waiting room. On Friday the staff would teach us what to do for Jamie. As we passed through the waiting room on our way out, we saw many parents still waiting to be told. For us, "Bloody Monday," the Institutes' term for this day of decision, was over.

Back in our hotel room we tried to sort out our impressions, but were too weary and confused to come to any conclusions. All I could do was write Jennifer two postcards, one from Mommy and Daddy and one from her brothers, then go to sleep.

Tuesday morning, in the waiting room, we tried to determine which families, if any, were missing. The rumor was that two families had been sent home. I noticed that most parents were more relaxed and friendly, and that the children with mobility seemed to gravitate more toward each other and away from parents. Parents were eager to share and compare histories and experiences of having a brain injured child, and the children were eager to find out who could talk or who had a doll or a truck that could be borrowed.

Again we spent most of the day waiting long periods between short appointments, and didn't leave until after 8:00 p.m. Besides two interesting but ancient movies about the Institutes' program, we saw seven people, ranging from a gruff old man who took our medical history yet again to an impersonal woman who measured the length and circumference of each of Jamie's limbs to a suave gentleman who talked very rapidly about the cost of the program. We finally saw an honest medical doctor who happened to be Glenn Doman's brother. After giving Jamie a brief examination, he quietly admitted that Jamie would probably always limp. He immediately looked as though he regretted having made that statement.

We went back to our hotel room feeling utterly discouraged. We got our two boys to sleep, and then Susan, Alden, and I sat on the beds and vented until midnight our disappointment and even anger over our two days of experiences at the Institutes for the Achievement of Human Potential. Our discussion boiled down to three complaints.

One reason for our disillusionment was that they had done nothing special to Jamie. I wasn't sure what our expectations had been—magic tests and space-age diagnostic machines or what—but certainly we had expected more than telling Jamie to look through a keyhole and reach in a bag and asking how many peas was he likely to eat with supper. We were medically oriented and the Institutes was functionally oriented.

Wait, wait, wait. That was our second gripe. We had wasted hours and hours doing nothing. That was totally against my efficient and compulsive nature. We had been told repeatedly that while we were idle, the staff was running. They were busy every minute and working until the wee hours making vital decisions about our child. But I was sure I could have organized it better. A lot of the brief chats could have been consolidated into one appointment. And much of what had to be explained could have been explained to the group as a whole instead of one family at a time. Were they trying to impress us with their complexity? And what was it that Glenn Doman had said about everyone smiling? We had noticed a distinct lack of warmth in most of the staff.

Finally, we were struck with disbelief when we studied the cost booklet. Three thousand dollars a year for the first two years! Payable in monthly installments of $250. After that the cost varied according to which of several options the parents chose. We had thought that the fee for this week (which was a reasonable $450) was the only fee until we came back again for reevaluation after three months. This $3000 came as a real shock, and we resented the fact that they waited until families were already there before disclosing this important factor. How could we afford this?

Alden wanted to pack up and go home. Though my confidence in the program had been severely shaken by the seemingly unsophisticated methods of assessment, the waiting, and the exorbitant cost, I still maintained enough belief to justify staying at least to hear Glenn Doman's lectures and what they would require Jamie to do on the program.

As we turned out the light and sank down onto our pillows, I silently asked myself if my inexorable belief in the Institutes, despite the valid protests of my husband and friend, was based on fact, or a desperate longing to help my beloved son, who I felt I had somehow afflicted with cerebral palsy. I had done it to him and I had to get rid of it. Though I, like many other mothers of hurt children, outwardly denied having guilt feelings, inwardly I knew that this was the last hope on earth for me as well as for Jamie.

14
Of Brain Injury and God

The great majority of children will do better than their parents had dared to hope.

Doman, 1974, p. 2

We had an extra-early, hurried breakfast at the cafe near the hotel on Wednesday morning because we had to drop Benjiman and Jamieson off at the waiting room at 8:25. Jamie would have some play time during the day, but also some work time while the staff determined what and how much of the program he was capable of participating in. I had originally thought that Susan would take care of Benjiman while Alden and I listened to Glenn Doman's lectures for two days. But we were told that Susan was welcome to attend the lectures, and they were willing to care for Benjiman in addition to Jamie. They would bring him to me at the lecture hall when he needed to be fed. They had also allowed Susan to eat lunch and dinner with us in the dining room at no charge.

There was a long line of parents and children in front of the angular building. Junior staff members dressed in overalls were slapping adhesive name tags on the backs of children and on their belongings, and taking the children one by one from the family at the head of the line, after which the parents, with notebooks in hand, left for the auditorium. We were quite friendly with several of the parents now and enjoyed some leisurely conversation with them in the lobby outside the auditorium.

There was the young couple who had a child with severe cerebral palsy. The mother was attractive and cordial, and was dressed in a black sheath and spiked heels. Her thinness bordered on frailty and I worried about her ability to carry her child around much longer and to do the strenuous program. There was a young foreign couple, whose baby had Down Syndrome. There were a mother and grandmother with a child that seemed hyperactive and disorganized. And there was another young couple who told us their child had been perfectly normal until the age of four when his throat had swollen until he could not breathe. The resulting brain damage had caused him to become blind.

Just before 9:00 a.m., we entered the auditorium. I was struck by its magnificence. I expected folding chairs and a portable chalkboard. What I saw was an oak paneled stage area with two matching lecterns, and ascending rows of long, highly polished tables, with microphones and plush swivel armchairs at each individual place. It was how I had always imagined the United Nations would look. There were even printed name cards at each place, giving the person's name and state or country of origin.

We were assigned to the third row. Susan and the other visitors were in the last row. In the back of that top row was a soundproof, glass-fronted little room where the translators sat. Those who did not speak English donned headphones that connected them to their translator.

As Alden and I began to set up our tape recorder and microphone, a staff member approached us and firmly forbade us to use the machine. The noise would be distracting, and all of Glenn Doman's lectures were available on tape at the bookstore in this same building.

At precisely 9:00 a.m., Glenn Doman strode onto the stage from a side door. There was an immediate hush in the room. He began by describing and defending the rules we were to observe for the next two days.

First, it was meant to be chilly in there. Research had shown that people scored 30 points higher on IQ tests in a cold room than in a warm room. Doman wanted us to be as alert as possible and to learn all that he taught us. And though he could not guarantee our child would win, "the exact degree to which you do not learn, your chances of winning will descend," he said.

Second, no questions were allowed from parents until a designated time, and visitors were never allowed to ask questions.

Last, there would be a ten-minute break at ten before each hour, and also a half-hour lunch break at 1:30 and a half-hour soup break at 6:00, signaled by a three-tone bell. When it sounded, we were to drop our pens and literally rush out to the lobby or outdoors to get the maximum benefit from the break, no matter if Doman was in the middle of a sentence. That was our time, not his. The end of the break would be signaled the same way, and we would have only a few seconds to return to our seats before the doors were closed and locked, to prevent disturbance during Glenn Doman's time. These rules had to be, he said, because it was imperative that we complete the agenda in the allotted time.

Doman went on to express his faith and respect for families, particularly mothers. He had discovered that in most cases it was the mother who had suspected something was wrong with her child long before a doctor. And it was mothers who worked with and made their children well on the program. The Institutes disagreed with Dr. X in Anywhere, USA, and so did we or we wouldn't be here. Standard tests only measured the disability of a brain injured child, and that was why the Institutes didn't use them. And it was easier to teach parents how to make their children well than it was to teach professionals because parents had less to unlearn than professionals, and most professionals were incapable of learning. Mothers, Doman went on, frequently sensed an underlying intelligence in their brain injured children. Most professionals had no use for these mothers. There was an unwritten law of professionals that said, "All mothers are idiots and the truth is not in them."

After only a few minutes of listening to Glenn Doman, I realized that he continually focused on the mothers' attachment to their children. "You've loved him nine months longer than Dad," "You have a deep emotional problem and you get up every morning with a heavy heart because your child is not well." He concluded his introductory remarks with, "Your family won't be well until your child is well." It was apparent that this man in whose control we would be for two days was a gifted and dynamic speaker and a master psychologist.

Doman's next subjects were what is brain injury and who is brain injured. Brain injury is in the brain. That is why exercises and braces did not work. We must treat the injury where it was: in the brain. The cause is always lack of oxygen to the brain, and it could occur at any point in one's life.

Who is brain injured? Everyone is brain injured to some degree. We all occupy a place on a continuum that ranges from death, coma, to being severely brain injured, moderately brain injured, mildly brain injured, hyperactive, unable to read, to being average, above average, superior, to ideal. There is no correlation, added Doman, between brain injury and intelligence. There is, however, a big correlation between brain injury and the ability to express intelligence. Many parents in the room nodded their heads in agreement with this.

How did Doman propose to treat a brain injured child, so that an individual could move up through the continuum? There were some basic assumptions that we would have to accept before the general statement of treatment could be understood.

First, we had to realize that brain growth is not predetermined and unalterable, but rather is a dynamic and ever changing process. It not only could be stopped or slowed, as by a brain injury, but it could also be speeded up, as when a brain injured child is made well.

Second, there is a law of physiology that says that function determines structure. As the athlete's biceps grow with use, so too does the brain grow with use, said Doman. Researchers had compared the brains of rats that lived in a deprived environment with the brains of rats that lived in an enriched environment, and found that the latter had significantly larger brains than the former. We could not look into the skulls of well kids or hurt kids made well, but we could assume by observing their mastery of sophisticated functions that their brains were larger than those of brain deficient or brain injured kids.

Third, we must remember that there is only one way that the brain receives information, through the five sensory pathways: visual, auditory, tactile, olfactory, and gustatory. The last two are of minor significance to humans, except in the case of coma or severe brain injury. The visual, auditory, and tactile senses are vital. They are the pathways that would allow us to grow the brain and to grow it at an accelerated rate.

Fourth, in order to assure that a message reaches the brain through either the visual, auditory, or tactile pathways, we must be sure that the message gets transmitted from one neuron to another on the way to the brain. The message would jump over the critical synapses (the spaces between neurons) only if it is strong enough. If we want to be sure that the message is strong enough to reach the brain, especially when the brain is injured, we must increase the frequency, intensity, and duration of the message.

The fifth principle was that after we successfully put information into the brain so that the brain may grow more rapidly, we need to give the owner of that brain plenty of opportunity to express motorically this new information.

These five assumptions were stated more concisely when Doman said, "All we do at the Institutes for the Achievement of Human Potential is to give a child visual, auditory, and tactile stimulation with increased frequency, intensity, and duration, along with unlimited opportunity to function, in full recognition of the orderly way in which the brain grows." He emphatically repeated this three times to be sure that the message was strong enough to cross the critical synapses on the way to our brains.

Several senior staff members had their turns on the stage that day and the next day to explain more fully what Glenn Doman meant by visual, auditory, and tactile stimulation, and by unlimited opportunity. We parents would find out at home what he meant by increased frequency, intensity, and duration.

The first person to relieve Glenn Doman on the stage was his daughter. She explained that the visual and auditory stimulation is given via the reading program. She declared that reading is a neurological function and not an academic subject. If we want to communicate to the brain the idea "flower," it makes no difference to the brain whether it sees the real thing or the word that stands for it, as long as the message gets there. If as adults talk to babies, the words could flash on the speaker's forehead, then babies would learn to read as quickly, as easily, and as early as they learn to talk. Since unfortunately we have no neon signs on our foreheads, babies take in the speaker's words only through one sensory pathway: the auditory pathway, and are therefore deprived of learning the visual representation of the word until years later when they aren't as eager to learn. This is a shame because reading is easy, reading is fun, reading is as vital as walking, reading creates intelligence, and reading actually physically "grows the brain".

Therefore, reading by using flashcards as a substitute for neon signs, is a part of every child's visual stimulation program at the Institutes, no matter how young. As the words are presented, the word is also spoken, thus providing auditory stimulation as well.

Children on the program receive tactile stimulation, the third part of the treatment definition, in the form of patterning. Patterning, or "closed brain surgery" as the staff liked to refer to it, is done on children who have no mobility or poor mobility because it sends the message over and over to the brain: This is how it feels to crawl, this is how it feels to creep. It is programming the brain, as one programs a computer, to crawl and creep.

Crawling and creeping are essential developmental stages. All children must crawl and creep. If either one of these stages is skipped or done poorly, the brain is not likely to function well in other tasks, both physical and intellectual. Crawling and creeping organizes the brain, and helps the person to move to the next level of brain development, where more functions are possible. That was the key statement for us and for Jamie. It explained why he would need to crawl and creep so much.

But one could not simply tell a brain injured child to crawl or creep. The brain must be programmed to crawl and to creep. Patterning is the method of programming the brain, telling it what coordinated movements were necessary. In fact, it would be okay to pattern a sleeping child because the message would still go to the brain.

The floor program provides the opportunity to express motorically what is received tactilely during patterning. This particular lecture was given by Glenn Doman's son. The Institutes was definitely a family affair. There was a look of alarm and disbelief on many parents' faces when he said that all nonwalkers must spend all day and all night prone on the floor! It had to be a smooth, hard, flat, clean, warm, and safe surface. No rugs. No beds. Arms, hands, legs, and feet must be bare for maximum tactile contact with the floor.

Much later, when questions were permitted, a couple asked if they must really get rid of the brand new crib for their baby. The answer was a serious, and emphatic "Yes." While on the floor, the child could not be supine, roll, sit up, or knee-walk. If he had a proclivity for any of these forbidden activities, various devices were demonstrated that could be strapped onto the child's back to absolutely prevent him from being able to do them. Nonwalkers would be picked up only for love, food, toileting, and administering other parts of the program. All this was to encourage the slightest movement forward, which of course would be immediately rewarded with lavish praise and maybe a favorite snack.

The floor is vital to every child's health, including well children, said young Doman. On the floor is where purposeful locomotion begins. Locomotion begins with simple crawling and leads, through a logical progression of increasingly sophisticated movement, to coordinated running. If a child can crawl 100 meters a day, then he is considered a confirmed crawler. If a child can crawl 330 meters a day in the cross pattern (opposite arm and leg moving forward at the same time, as opposed to the homologous pattern in which the arm and leg on the same side move forward at the same time), then he is ready to creep. If he can creep 400 meters a day, then he is a confirmed creeper. If he can creep 1.6 kilometers (one mile) a day, then he is ready to stand with support. If he can do 1,000 ladder walks (walking while holding onto a low overhead ladder for support) a day, he is ready to walk alone. If he can walk 1.6 kilometers a day, then he is a confirmed walker. If he can walk 1.6 kilometers a day in less than 20 minutes, then he is ready to run. And if he can run 4.8 kilometers (three miles) a day in less than 30 minutes, then he has reached a goal known at the Institutes as physical excellence.

Another lecture dealt with providing an optimum internal environment for brain growth through masking, nutrition, and liquid balance. It was discovered that brain injured children do not breathe well, so their brains never get all the oxygen they need. Breathing carbon dioxide for a minute activates an automatic reflex which causes blood vessels to dilate, and makes one breathe more deeply and slowly. In this way, more oxygen gets to the brain after that minute of breathing carbon dioxide. This is the Institutes' justification for masking. Glenn Doman even confided that he had regularly masked himself every day since his 60th birthday, with the intention of reducing his chances of having a stroke.

The second way to control the internal environment of the brain so that it might grow better is through liquid balance. Hippocrates observed many centuries ago that injured brains are moist. Now it is known that as the liquid in and around the brain is decreased, the amount of oxygenated blood that can circulate in the brain is increased. Therefore there is an ideal amount of fluid that should be consumed by each child each day. Unless there is a hot spell, or the child has diarrhea, vomiting, or fever, it is not the eight glasses that we have always heard about. The ideal is much less than half of that for most children.

The third way to control the internal environment of the brain is through nutrition. A proper balance of high quality natural foods and supplemental vitamins and minerals is prescribed for all children on the program. Sugar, artificial colors and flavors, processed foods, additives, and preservatives are not allowed. Improper diet could produce seizures or coma. Proper diet could produce "abundant health, superb function, and robust structure."

I have greatly compressed what took two full days to present. There were other, lesser lectures comparing programming the brain to programming a computer, on treating coma victims, on the different institutes that make up the Institutes for the Achievement of Human Potential and their individual objectives and treatment principles, and on the Developmental Profile that is the main tool of each institute. It was pointed out many times that the methods used by the Institutes are beneficial to the well child too, and in fact would make the well child superior. A large part of the Institutes' research and applications does involve normal children, we were told. Despite the fact that much of what was taught was a repeat of what we had read in Doman's book, it was never boring. Doman had an entertaining or moving story to embellish every point or principle he was trying to convey, and this human factor made understanding and retention of the material easier.

Many times during the two days when we hurriedly left the auditorium at the sound of the bells for our ten-minute break and retreat to warmth, I would find a staff member in her coveralls holding my crying baby in the lobby. I would then go into the translators' area to feed Benji. I sat with the three translators, all jabbering at once in Spanish, Italian, and Japanese, and put on my own set of headphones and listened to the speaker. At the next break, there would be someone waiting to take a burped and sleepy baby back to the waiting room in the other building. I never missed a word. It was a smooth system.

During Glenn Doman's closing remarks, at 9:00 on Thursday, he stated that families exist to divide time up unevenly. It is okay to give more time to the one who needs it. If we decide to divide up our time evenly within the family because we love the well kid so much, then when that well child reaches adulthood she would consider it no favor that we destroyed her brain injured sibling for her sake. Or if we decide to put the hurt kid in an institution, all we would be doing is teaching the well kid where to put us when we grow old.

Glenn Doman was a skilled salesman, and we were aware of his skill. That was, after all, what he was doing—selling his program. Doman's objective was to make our children well, but he was careful to say that he did not guarantee to make anyone's child well. The only thing he did guarantee was "blood, sweat, and tears." He said that he would throw out anyone who fell behind. He said that kids were literally dying to get in and that no family could occupy a place on the roster who did not do all of the program exactly as instructed. He told of a family who, after many months of waiting, had recently arrived on a Sunday night for the week of evaluations, and their child died in the night at the hotel. The family still stayed for the two days of lectures in order to learn what could have helped their child.

The very last thing that Glenn Doman did was to take out a Bible and read from The Book of Revelations, Chapter 3, verses 7 through 13. This told of a message from God to, of all places, the church of Philadelphia:

This is the message from one who is holy and true, who holds the key..., who opens so that none can close, who closes so that none can open... You have followed my teaching and been faithful to me. I have opened a door before you, which no one can close. Listen! ...Because you have kept my order to be patient, I will also keep you safe from the time of trouble... Keep safe what you have, so that no one will rob you of your victory prize. I will make him who is victorious a pillar in the temple... If you have ears, then listen to what the spirit says to the churches!

As he closed the Bible and dismissed us with a silent nod, I wondered what Glenn Doman's middle initial was.

15
Of Brain Injury and Brainwashing

Some medics and teachers see the concept of neurological organization as a possible breakthrough.

Bird, 1967, p. 28

The discussion that took place in our hotel room late Thursday night was quite different from the discussion that had taken place late Tuesday night. We were all full of renewed hope and eager to begin a unique program that just might work. Maybe we (and all the others) really could "fix our kids," as Glenn Doman had repeatedly phrased our privilege. We were so animated and jubilant at the prospect that Jamie complained he couldn't sleep. We lowered our voices, but did not discontinue our conversation, indeed our celebration, even as we brushed our teeth and changed into our bedclothes.

We reviewed our notes of two days and could find nothing untrue or objectionable. The most appealing aspect was that nothing about the program could hurt Jamie. There wouldn't be any operations or medications. The only place it would hurt was in our wallet, and we would somehow bear that. We shuddered to think that we had almost left. Our sleep that night was as sound as our beliefs.

Doman and his staff had been very convincing. His theories were simple and logical. But his subtle control of the group with his bells and rules and calculated remarks had not gone unnoticed by us. He told us that one family in our group, and only one, would not be back for the reevaluation in three months. Everyone had silently vowed not be that one highly visible family who would be deemed a failure by all the others. We felt that the fact that we were intelligent enough and perceptive enough to recognize these pressures meant that we couldn't possibly be influenced by them. It was Doman's wisdom that had won us back, not his wiles.

We ate breakfast Friday morning at our usual spot. Benjiman was having his breakfast too, so I had to ask Alden to spread the butter on my muffin for me because I, like Jamie, could not accomplish that task with my one free hand. As we ate, we heard on the television some tragic news for America. President Carter's daring rescue attempt the night before of the United States citizens held hostage since November in the American

Embassy in Iran had failed. Helicopters had crashed, lives had been lost, and the surviving forces were retreating. It was a sad morning for the families of the still detained hostages, and for Carter's reelection campaign.

We didn't break our necks to be punctual for our first appointment of the day. We checked in with the receptionist in the waiting room, and then sat down with our friends to wait. The waiting didn't seem so much drudgery as it had on previous days, partially because we were accustomed to it and anticipated it, and partially because of the contagious zeal that now existed among the parents for Doman's program, even though it had not yet been fully revealed to us, nor even tried by anyone except us. Undoubtedly, some of the parents in our group considered Jamie a walking advertisement for the program. They disregarded the fact that his degree of brain injury was significantly less than that exhibited by some of the other children in our group. There was a strong need, on their part as well as ours, to attribute at least some of his ability to the five-week preliminary program we had done with him prior to coming to Philadelphia.

There was an unverified rumor among the parents that all staff members at the Institutes were required to crawl, creep, and brachiate a certain amount each day. We saw them all in coveralls at one time or another, and there was indeed a crawling, creeping, and brachiating course on the grounds, located apart from the random ladders that seemed to be for us. We observed very young nonbrain injured children, part of the Evans Thomas Institute and the Better Baby Institute, using it, but we never saw a staff member do anything on it besides supervise the young participants.

We learned during the lectures that the Institutes was divided into three main parts—the Institute for the Achievement of Physical Excellence, the Institute for the Achievement of Intellectual Excellence, and the Institute for the Achievement of Physiological Excellence. Staff members for each institute could be identified by the colors of their blazers and pants or skirts. Those attached to the Institute for the Achievement of Physical Excellence wore black blazers and gray pants or skirts, those of the Institute for the Achievement of Intellectual Excellence wore tan blazers and black pants and skirts, and those of the Institute for the Achievement of Physiological Excellence wore maroon blazers and camel pants or skirts.

Our first appointment was with a black blazer, Physical Excellence. She took us to a little room upstairs that contained her desk and a patterning table. She handed us a blue sheet that had blanks for the recipient to fill in as to the type of pattern to be done, number (frequency) done each day (duration), amount of time for each one (intensity), and the number of people required to do it. We were to do eight five-minute cross patterns a day, using three adults. I cringed when she warned that patternings must be spaced at least a half an hour apart, and ideally more than that. I had already known I would need more volunteers to cover Wednesday, the day

I had no volunteers, but now it appeared that I would need to create more sessions for every day to minimally meet the spacing requirements and the increase in the total number of patterns from six to eight. I could not do it with just two volunteers a day in one session. I would now need to ask people to sit in my house for three and a half hours. I could not do that. I figured that eight cross patterns could be reasonably done in three separate one-hour sessions. But it would triple my need for help.

The lady in the black blazer also handed us several white sheets with drawings of exactly how to build a patterning table, and drawings of how to move the child on that table. She told us to sprinkle a little corn starch on the vinyl if there was too much friction, due to sweat or other dampness, when moving Jamie's limbs. Next, she had us demonstrate how we patterned Jamie. She gave her approval and, as we had no further questions, sent us back to the waiting room.

Soon a maroon blazer, Physiological Excellence, came looking for us. From her we received two yellow sheets on the rules of masking and how to care for the masks. Again we filled in the blanks—80 times (frequency), at seven minute intervals (duration), for 60 seconds at a time (intensity). We were told to use five or six masks at a time, rotating their use all day so that one could dry out before it was used again. As soon as one got ripped or too dirty, it should be discarded. Our three-month supply of masks could be picked up in the main office at our convenience when we went in to pay our bill for the week. We demonstrated our proficiency at masking and went back to the waiting room.

As usual, there was no posted agenda, and we had no idea when we were to be seen by whom. We had one more meeting with a black blazer, one with a maroon blazer, one with a tan blazer, and an overview with our advocate, a total of six meetings for the day. Two with Physical Excellence, one with Intellectual Excellence, two with Physiological Excellence, and one with our less-than-warm advocate. At no time were we given pre-written instructions specifically for Jamie. It was always general sheets of information with blanks that we filled in as they dictated.

Our final appointment with the Institute for the Achievement of Physiological Excellence concerned nutrition and vitamin supplements. No salty foods were to be given because liquids must be limited to 20 ounces a day. Jamie was not a heavy drinker so I knew this would be no problem. No sugar, no white flour, no artificial colors, and no preservatives were to be given. I had already eliminated as much as possible of the latter three from our diet for two years. Though Jamie and Jennifer were not addicted to sweets, and I always refused the lollipop at the bank and at the doctor's, I did still occasionally allow the kids to have jelly, maple syrup, ice cream, and other desserts. These things must go, said the maroon jacket.

Jamie must consume 45 to 50 grams of protein in a day, one third of

which must be ingested in the morning so as to have sustained energy for
the rest of the day's physical program. We were handed a sheet that told the
protein content of most common foods. In addition, Jamie must have 22 IUs
of vitamin E a day, 5,000 IUs of vitamin A a day, 500 milligrams of vitamin
C four times a day (or once every hour if sick), and a tablespoon a day of a
particular vitamin B-complex preparation. The entire family should follow
the same regimen, including the baby in reduced doses. All these vitamins
could be purchased at a discount at the bookstore on the grounds. During
our lunch break we went to the bookstore and spent over $200 on dis-
counted vitamins, and on books others had written in support of the
Institutes.

Our second appointment with a person wearing a black blazer was a
long one. The young man took us downstairs to tell us how much crawling,
creeping, and brachiating Jamie should do daily. We sat in a room that was
like a workout room, with several mats and eight overhead ladders. He
handed us the now familiar blue sheets, and Alden filled in the blanks while
I fed Benjiman. Jamie's crawling goal was to do 880 yards, or ½ mile a day.
This goal would be reached gradually, beginning by doing 30 yards
(intensity) five times (frequency) every day (duration) the first week. He
would then work up to 50 yards at a time five times a day by week three, 100
yards four times a day by week five, and 220 yards four times a day by week
seven. And Jamie's creeping goal was to do two miles a day. Creeping was
easier and faster than crawling, so four times as much was required. Again,
this goal would be reached gradually, beginning with 50 yards (intensity)
eight times (frequency) every day (duration) the first week, working up to
100 yards at a time six times a day by week three, 200 yards five times a day
by week five, 440 yards four times a day by week seven, and 880 yards four
times a day by week nine.

I watched the figures that Alden was writing as rapidly as they were
dictated and tried to figure out how it all related to the amount that Jamie
had already been doing every day. We had measured his crawling and
creeping time, but not distance. How far was it around that patterning table
and how many times did he go around it? I had a disturbing conviction that
his crawling hadn't anywhere near approached a half mile, nor his creeping
two miles. Sometimes Jamie barely moved. It was his nature to be slow. I
would either have to speed him up or be prepared to stay up with him all
night.

The black jacket made several more points concerning crawling and
creeping. Though no maximum or minimum time limit was suggested, all
crawling and creeping was to be timed and accurately recorded for the
interim and revisit reports. Elbow and knee pads were permitted. Jamie,
who had shown no reaction to the unknown numbers that had been reeled
off, now grinned with relief. We were to measure several indoor and

outdoor tracks, and while Jamie could creep on any surface, he had to crawl only on a smooth, hard, flat surface. I was silently thankful when our instructor indicated that since Jamie could already move and walk he would not have his bed taken away from him and be required to sleep, as well as crawl, on a smooth, hard, flat surface, as Glenn Doman had threatened was in store for some during his lectures.

Without further time for questions or contemplation of crawling and creeping, the young man in the black blazer moved on to brachiation. Though brachiating had not been mentioned in the lectures as one of the procedures that organized the brain, it was now explained to us that its main value was to grow a child's chest and to improve his respiratory structure. In other words, to breathe better and to thereby insure that oxygen got to the brain. Only an oxygenated brain could grow. In Jamie's particular case, brachiating was also intended to improve his hand function.

The man adjusted the height of one of the ladders so that Jamie could barely reach it standing stretched out and on tiptoe. Fifty-one inches off the floor was right. Then he had Jamie hold onto 1-inch dowels, ³/₄-inch dowels, and ¹/₂-inch dowels. For Jamie's hand size and grasping ability, ³/₄-inch dowels were best. Alden had made our ladder with 1-inch dowels. He would have to redo it when we got home. Jamie was to walk under the ladder at this height holding onto the rungs, 20 times a day for the first week, 30 the second, 40 the third, and 50 from the fourth week on. This was the precursor to brachiating with his feet off the ground. The ultimate goal was to brachiate 30 single trips a day across the ladder with or without support. For this brachiating, the ladder should be raised high enough for an adult to walk under it and hold onto Jamie's waist, giving him just enough support for him to be successful, and swinging him just enough to teach him to use his body's momentum to go from rung to rung.

So in addition to the daily ladder walks, Jamie was to hang, without moving, 20 times for one minute every day for the first week, hang 30 times for one minute the second week, hang 15 times and brachiate the length of the ladder 10 times the third week, brachiate 20 times a day the fourth week, brachiate 25 times a day the fifth week, and brachiate 30 times across the ladder every day by the sixth week.

I silently resigned myself to developing terrific arm muscles as I carried Jamie across the 12-foot ladder 30 times a day. He could never do it alone. Couldn't they see what was wrong with this child?

We were warned that Jamie's hands would be quite sore, and in fact, possibly raw from all this. But we must never use cream or lotion as those only soften the hands and make them more vulnerable to further sores. It was best to wipe his hands twice a day with alcohol and soon tough callouses would form to protect his hands.

Our instructor casually mentioned that our baby, though not brain injured, should spend his days on the floor, and not in an infant seat or walker, in order to allow him to crawl naturally and creep as much as possible before walking. We assured him that the infant seat and the walker had been thrown out after we had read Glenn Doman's book, and that with the program we had just been assigned I would seldom have time to hold the baby, so he was destined to be on the floor a great deal of the time. Since he had brought up the benefits of the program to other kids, I chose that moment to ask about Jennifer's crossed eye. He said that crawling, creeping, and brachiating done in the same amount as was assigned to Jamie, and done without her glasses on, would definitely cure her strabismus.

We went back to the waiting room in a daze to peruse our blue sheets. Patterning, masking, and nutrition took no time or effort. But this was different. Crawling and creeping and brachiating could take hours and hours and hours.

By now it was midafternoon and, as I looked up from my papers, I suddenly became aware of a new phenomenon in the waiting room. Parents were not socializing with other parents. They were absorbed with trying out the new techniques on their children. Several were staring fixedly at their watches as they timed a masking, others were for the first time using the patterning tables for patterning, some were on the floor creeping with their kids, and still others were studying their instruction sheets of assorted colors.

We had one more complex set of instructions to receive. A vivacious young woman in a tan blazer and black skirt, Intellectual Excellence, took us to her office to tell us how to teach our son to read. I filled in the blanks on white sheets as she explained that Jamie should be presented with 100 words a day. These 100 words should be printed in large red print on flash cards, and they should be divided into ten categories of ten words each. Each category should be shown twice a day for a total of 20 reading sessions. She gave us a list of vocabulary suggestions—colors, fruits, vehicles, and so on. The most extraordinary requirement was that each of these 20 lessons was to last only ten seconds!

I must never ask him what a word was. I was to say the word as I showed it, and flip through the pack of ten cards as fast as I could, and then return immediately to creeping or whatever. I was to write the word lightly in pencil on the reverse where it would act as a cue to me so that I would not be slowed down by trying to see the front side of the card as I held it 18 inches from Jamie's face. Each day, after the first ten days, I must remove one pack of ten and add a new pack of ten. Each individual word was therefore shown just 20 times, two times a day for ten days, one second each time, before it was retired.

After two weeks of this, I was to begin showing Jamie couplets. He must see five categories of three related couplets twice a day, again each session lasting only ten seconds or less. I was to use retired single words in combinations, like "red truck," "blue car," and "yellow bus." Those three couplets, written on three separate cards, constituted one category and was shown ten times, twice a day for five days, before being exchanged for three new couplets.

Also, after two weeks of single words, I was to begin putting together random short sentences for Jamie to read three times a day. And I was to read to him once a day one homemade book of five or six pages, with one sentence per page of 1-inch print. Articles did not need to be taught, just used. Each book was to be used for one week, and then retired, and a new one presented for the following week.

It was impossible to thoroughly absorb all these instructions while sitting in her office. I knew it would be clearer when I had studied it and actually done it for a few days. I had used flash cards with Jennifer and with Jamieson; I just hadn't done it with such speed or organization. Two things were immediately apparent. This was a unique teaching method that no public school system was likely to sanction, and this was going to require a tremendous amount of preparation on our part. There were no preprinted word cards or booklets available at the Institutes. Our instructor insisted that was not feasible because each child's native language varies, and each family's surroundings and unique experiences, used as the source of the homemade stories, also varies. The parents are therefore best suited to making up the word categories and the stories.

When we had no further questions and were about to leave, she offered one more suggestion. I should begin making word cards for Benjiman as soon as possible. When I changed his diaper I should hold up a card that said "diaper" and when he looked at his sister I should hold up a card that said "Jennifer." He could of course learn to read before he learned to talk.

We returned to the waiting room for what turned out to be our last wait of the week. It was almost 5:00 p.m. and the number of families still present had dwindled to about half a dozen. We were shortly summoned by our advocate, who had made himself scarce through the week and who had certainly made no effort to get to know us.

He sat at his desk and reviewed Jamie's program, a complete copy of which he had before him, with all the blanks filled in. He handed us a bulky midterm report and end of term report and looked toward but not at us. He then blandly warned us that we must do everything exactly as instructed. He told us we must keep accurate daily records, half of which would be sent in with the interim report and the rest to be brought with us at the revisit, that we must make a chart for Jamie to understand what was expected of him on a daily basis and what rewards he could earn for meeting his goals, that all the goals were only minimums and that if we could exceed any of the goals we would be helping Jamie to get well that much faster, that we must send him a picture of Jamie using his ladder by May 15 (to prove that we had in fact built one?), and that above all we must keep smiling and make the program fun for Jamieson.

We went to the receptionist's office to have holes punched in our stack of rainbow colored papers that we had collected so that they could be neatly preserved in the notebook they had "given" us, said our goodbyes and good-lucks to the few parents we passed in the waiting room, paid our bill and picked up Jamie's masks and our diploma in another building. We declined the last supper in the dining room in favor of a meal in different surroundings, and went back to our hotel for a good night's sleep before the long trip home early the next morning.

If Benjamin could describe the passengers in the car with him that morning, I wondered if he would find a total of one brain injured child and three brainwashed adults.

16
Getting Ready Again

There are armies of neighbors and friends waiting to help.

Melton, 1972, p. 168

Everything seemed a jumble to us. There was so much new information to absorb that I felt disorganized. After the drive home I worked Saturday evening and Sunday to turn our pile of instructions into a clear and orderly daily agenda and weekly progression. I had to know what I was doing before I could do it. After tiresome rereading and charting, it finally made sense to me.

The next steps were to organize the house to meet the requirements of the program, to buy certain materials for implementing the program, and then to actually try the program on Jamie.

We had to create and measure new paths for creeping and crawling. Since there were 3520 yards in two miles, and since it was only ten yards around the patterning table, it would take 352 trips around the table to reach two miles! That would surely drive Jamie berserk. So we measured out an interesting 50-yard course upstairs that went around the living room, down the hall, in and out of the bathroom and all the bedrooms, and back to the living room. Eighteen consecutive times on that course would be 900 yards, a little over the 880-yard goal that was eventually to be accomplished four times a day. I recalled our advocate's warning that more was better.

With summer coming and a beautiful pool in our back yard, there was no way we could be expected to stay cooped up indoors. We needed an outdoor creeping and crawling course as well. The fence around the pool area was 50 feet on each side. There was a brick patio and lawn furniture along one side. The other three sides were grassy. If Jamie started creeping in one corner of the pool area, followed the fence for three sides, and then turned around and came back to his starting point, he would have covered 100 yards. Creeping that course nine consecutive times would equal 900 yards, again a little over the 880-yard goal that was eventually to be accomplished four times a day.

Crawling was to be done only on a smooth, hard surface. The less friction the easier the movement. That eliminated most of the house. But we had linoleum in the kitchen. I visually surveyed the kitchen. There was the large refrigerator and brick wall containing the wall oven at one end. At the far end was the round, glass-topped table with the large spool for a base. There were no obstacles down the center. I got out my yardstick. If Jamie started at the refrigerator and crawled to the opposite end of the kitchen around the table, and then back to the refrigerator, that would be ten yards. It was not a long, interesting route, but it was the best I could do. If he crawled 22 consecutive times around the table and back, it would equal exactly the 220 yards that Jamie was to do four times a day.

We also needed an outdoor crawling course in addition to the indoor course. But where to do it was the question. The paved driveway and the brick patio were both too rough, and the grass was forbidden. Alden thought of a solution. He would buy five sheets of 8' x 4' masonite, nail them together, and lay them on top of the grass along one 50 foot side of the fence around the pool area. It was the same strip that was the first leg of the creeping course. The total round trip length of the smooth, hard, flat surface would be 80 feet. A few feet would be lost as Jamie started in the prone position and as he flopped over at the far end because there wouldn't be enough width to execute a proper U-turn. So he would call it 75 feet, or 25 yards, per round trip, a figure which would also be more amenable to calculations of distance. Crawling nine round trips on this outdoor course would equal 225 yards, only a little over the required 200 yards that Jamie was to do four times a day.

All that remained in adapting our house to this strange new program was to be able to do Jamie's ladder work and cross patterning outdoors as well. Alden would construct another ladder in the pool area, in addition to changing the rung size on the one already downstairs, and we would convert our picnic table to a patterning table. It wouldn't be as sturdy or as high or as wide as the official one, but with a little foam padding and vinyl covering tacked on, it wouldn't be bad.

We made a shopping list and did our errands that Sunday afternoon. We didn't intend to waste any time. "Time is the enemy", Glenn Doman had said often. Alden took Jamie with him to get the building materials.

I took Jennifer and Benjiman with me and headed for the mall. In a department store I bought a stopwatch. Though there was no specified time limit for each stint of creeping and crawling, it was all supposed to be carefully timed and recorded on blue forms. We had a feeling that speed, though not required, would be essential to accomplishing the goals. The watch was also needed to accurately time maskings when we would be outdoors or upstairs, away from the schoolhouse clock with the sweeping second hand in the therapy room downstairs. I already had a bell timer to remind me when the patterning was done or when it was time to mask again, but I bought another one just in case it broke or I lost it. Next, I bought two red magic markers and ten large sheets of white poster board to cut up into word cards and storybook pages, a three-ring notebook to keep the stories in, and two small spiral notebooks to make a daily record for transferring to the midterm and final reports. In the same store, I also bought three grocery counters. They were little plastic clickers on which one was supposed to register the amount of each purchase in dollars and cents up to $99.99, so as not to exceed one's budget. I planned to use one for the number of yards crawled, one for the number of yards crept, and one for the number of maskings completed in the dollars place and number of ladder walks and brachiates in the cents place. Everything had to be counted as well as timed, and there was no sense depending on memory. How clever I was to think of this easy method of tabulation. A feeling of smug efficiency swept over me, replacing my earlier feeling of befuddlement.

My next stop was at a sports store for two sets of elbow and knee pads, one for Jamie and one for Jennifer. Then I went to the Vision Center to pick up Jennifer's new glasses. The lenses were thicker than I had expected and the big round frames seemed gawkier than I recalled them. I told her they looked lovely, and secretly hoped it would not be long before I could stow them in the attic next to the unneeded casts. My last stop was at the fabric store. I bought an expensive six-foot piece of three-inch foam and two and a half yards of black vinyl.

After supper and after putting three little children to bed, I prepared another ad for the newspaper to recruit more volunteers. Ideally, I needed 16 different people every weekday, or a total of 80, to come two at a time, for five minutes, eight different times a day. That wasn't possible, given where we lived and my aversion to strangers. We decided we needed only five people a day, two who would come together for 1¼ hours and do three cross patterns, two more who would come together at a later hour to do three more cross patterns with me, and a fifth person to come when Alden was home from work to do the last two cross patterns. That meant I had to have 19 more people than the four I already had, two of whom were already coming twice a week. Should I aim for 21 more people so those two did not have to do double duty?

We concluded that families with brain injured children who lived in busy city apartment complexes, where there was a never ending source of patterners who could just pop in at a moment's notice, fared better on the Institutes' program than a family with a brain injured child who lived in a rural area where one could barely see one's nearest neighbors, whom one hardly knew anyway. On the other hand, how did city-bound apartment dwellers find space to do all that creeping and crawling?

While we were discussing this predicament, I was making lists of potential reading words, grouped into categories of ten, and Alden was cutting each of the ten pieces of cardboard into 24 3" x 12" reading cards. That yielded 24 piles of ten cards each, which, at the rate of one new category of ten related words a day, was less than a month's supply of cards. And that didn't even include the cardboard that I would need for couplets and books. I made a mental note to call around to various stores to find the least expensive source of cardboard. We also prepared a dozen new masks for use. The elastic string coming out of each side of the masks had to be knotted together so that the mask could be readily slipped on and off Jamie's head, the two little holes on top of the mask had to be taped over to minimize the entrance of air, and the two ends of the metal nose piece had to be bent in such a way as to prevent their poking a hole in the thin plastic through repeated use.

Though there was much more to do, we retired early that night in hopes of overcoming a week's worth of mental and physical exhaustion, and of being fresh for tomorrow's responsibilities—both Alden's at the shipyard and mine at home.

For three days, Monday, Tuesday, and Wednesday, I experimented with Jamie's new program. For those days I did not keep any records of his attempts or accomplishments. I needed to figure out what sequences afforded the smoothest transitions and which things fit in best in the time between cross patterns while I had volunteers in and had to keep to a schedule. Should he brachiate and then crawl, or should he creep and then brachiate, or didn't it matter? Should he do the things that he hated most first, and then do the things that he was better able to tolerate, or, in the interest of speed, should he do what he liked first when he was fresh, and then drag through what he disliked? And just what was there in this program that he liked?

A lot of time was lost in those first days because I had to describe our experiences at the Institutes to our volunteers. They were eager to know all they could, and my enthusiasm was mostly genuine, but also a little calculated in order to maintain their belief in the program, and thus their willingness to continue coming. All they knew they got from me. It was imperative that I be a good teacher. Cora Jo responded to my plea for more volunteers. She said she would get her best friend, Helen, to come, and that her next door neighbor, Darlene, belonged to a woman's group at church and would surely be willing to help. I also became bold one night and called five of my neighbors to ask for help.

First, I called Judi, not really a neighbor, but a good friend. She had cared for Jennifer while we were in Philadelphia and had already offered to help. It was an easy call. Next I called my nearest neighbor and closest friend on the street, Susan Monday. I had already told her about the program. She too had already offered to help, as long as I wouldn't mind her bringing her own three children and the three or four or five or six others she babysat daily. Next, I called Barbara, who had been our first regular babysitter for Jamie. She now had a two-year old son of her own, and was still living nearby. Then I called Bonnie, who had also been one of our best babysitters, and was now married and had a one-year old daughter. I called Marj, whom I had seen only twice since she had married the single fellow across the street. She had a baby only a few weeks older than Benjiman. I made a sixth call, to Mary, a casual acquaintance who lived in the next town, because I thought she would be receptive. I knew there would be a Catch-22 in asking her—she was an Avon Lady.

I felt guilty because I was asking for more than a one-time commitment, and because the request—help for a disabled child—made it difficult for a person to gracefully refuse. But I was desperate. Judi, Susan, Barbara, Bonnie, Marj, and Mary all said they would come at the times I assigned them. And even better, Susan Monday said she would come twice, and she and Judi both offered to substitute any time someone else couldn't make it.

Thursday, May 1, 1980 was the day that I considered to be the official starting day of the official program. I had a shortage of volunteers, but with the new ad I hoped to have that problem alleviated by the following week. We had to get started. I dated the top of the first page of one of my tiny spiral notebooks and wrote "Day 1." On separate lines I wrote Jamie's seven different tasks that I needed to keep close count of: masking, walking, brachiating, crawling, creeping, cross patterning, and reading. In the space beside each I would write the required goals for that day, and beside that, how many or how much of each he actually accomplished. Ideally, the two numbers would match—goals should be met. The goals that I wrote down for brachiating, walking, creeping, and crawling were for week number seven because we were too experienced in the program to begin at ground zero. Only in reading would he be at the beginning. At the bottom of my notebook was a space to record questions or thoughts or observations, and I imagined I would fill that up easily every day.

I was now totally prepared and organized for carrying out the program. Jamie came home from kindergarten at 11:00, and I met him at the door with a mask as usual. I moved the kitchen chairs out of the way, and then I had him crawl 220 yards, from the refrigerator around the table and back, 22 times, while I fixed lunch. Alden delivered Jennifer at 11:45, just as Jamie was finishing his crawling, and then had to hurry back to the shipyard. I fed the kids lunch, and at 12:00 Barbara and Mary came for their three patterns. All went well, and Jamie did a considerable amount of work between patterns.

Bonnie and Marj came at three. I put Benjiman on the floor under a mobile I had hung off one end of the patterning table and hoped he would be amused. Bonnie put her toddler daughter beside the toy box. Marj put her infant son on the floor under the ladder. I had to instruct Bonnie and Marj in the fine art of closed brain surgery, or patterning, as they previously had only received a telephone description. As soon as I set the timer for five minutes and the three of us were rhythmically moving Jamie on the table, all three babies began to cry. Jennifer, who might have quieted at least one, was upstairs and out of earshot. We continued to cross pattern, but at a tempo that matched the wailing around us. When the bell sounded, each mother let go of Jamie and ran to console her own child. Soon it was quiet except for muffled maternal murmurs, and an occasional pitiful sob. The next two cross patterns were equally as distressing as the first, as the three children cried wholeheartedly when put down. Bonnie's little girl could creep and always found her way to her mother's legs. She pulled herself up and spent the five minutes pulling at Bonnie's jeans and screaming, completely perplexed as to why her mother would not pay any attention to her. I was amazed when Bonnie and Marj were leaving to hear them both offer to come on Tuesdays, as well as Thursdays, to fill another time slot for me! I would have been less amazed if they had declined to come again at all.

Alden got home at 4:30, and started supper while I continued to work with Jamie downstairs. Six o'clock came and went and Pattianne never showed up.

Benjiman remained fussy all evening, and not many of Jamie's quotas were met. My notebook looked like this at the end of that first day after entering the totals from my grocery clickers.

Day 1, May 1, 1980

Goals	Frequency	Intensity	Amount
masking	60	1 min.	50
walking	50		15
brachiating	25		10
crawling	4	220 yd.	20, 25, 30 min.
creeping	4	440 yd.	20, 18, 22, 25 min.
patterning	8	5 min.	6
reading	20	10 sec.	20

I circled the best times of crawling and creeping to be entered on the official report form later. The only goals that we met on Day 1 were reading and nutrition. And everything but patterning and masking was to be increased the following week. After making a few notes at the bottom of the page describing the events of the day, I went to bed at 9:00 p.m., totally exhausted and defeated.

Day 2 went more smoothly. Benjiman was back to his good-natured self. Judi, who came at noon to pattern, took Jennifer home with her to play with her daughter. Pattianne showed up for her time, and I had Jamie do 100 yards of crawling in the kitchen before he even went to school in the morning. We met all the goals for the day except in ladder work. Walking 50 times under the ladder was time-consuming, and then raising the ladder and carrying Jamie while he tried to brachiate 25 times was also time-consuming, as well as back-breaking. We could not yet reach those goals.

In pursuing these goals, Jamie was enduring some battle scars. He had the expected blisters on his hands, which I dutifully wiped clean with alcohol. His arms ached from supporting some of his own weight while brachiating. His toes ached from stretching while walking under the almost too high ladder. I had heard it said that one had to be a physical wreck before one could become a physical specimen. Jamie was at the wreck stage, and we hoped the specimen stage was not far off. Fortunately, his elbows and knees were protected now while crawling and creeping by elbow and knee pads. He didn't need any more pain.

Friday night, and over the weekend, I got four calls in response to my second ad for volunteers, two of which got me a firm commitment. One was a pleasant surprise—it was Alden's cousin Anita, who lived 30 minutes away but whom we seldom saw. She wanted to come for two whole afternoons each week, participating in four of the 15 patterning sessions during weekdays. The other new caller who signed up was a woman named Jane.

Cora Jo also called that weekend to say that her friend Helen could come with her on Monday, and could her old partner Etta possibly come at a different time. Cora Jo's neighbor Darlene called to say that she and four other women from her church group, Diana, Winona, Dot, and Piera, could come. And Lynne, who was the classroom aide in Jamie's kindergarten, and who knew about Jamie's new program because she was a friend of Susan Monday's, called to say she would like to help too.

I considered it a miracle that I had all 25 spots filled! My only problem was finagling with the schedule so that everyone could come on her preferred day or with her favorite partner. I spent hours and hours getting it finalized.

As I was patting myself on the back for this accomplishment, I realized that Alden too deserved recognition for his weekend work. Though the pool was still covered for the winter, and the days were still cool, he had prepared the pool area for the days when we would want to be outside to do the program. He had tacked the foam and vinyl onto the picnic table and had built the outdoor ladder in the pool area and secured it to the fence. We joked about the fact that the rungs of this new ladder had already become a favorite perching spot for our numerous back yard birds, and were covered with white droppings. "I don't mind building a ladder to cure my son, but I do object to building a toilet for all the birds in the neighborhood!" lamented the weary carpenter.

Alden's final, and most exasperating, job of the weekend was screwing together the masonite crawl course. The newly completed outdoor crawl course covered up a long stretch of grass that we had finally (after two years of failure) coaxed into growing. The young grass would die for a good cause, we declared.

17
What Number Am I On?

This is not the kind of childhood Mother and Daddy had planned for you, son.
Melton, 1968, p. 167

I became obsessed with numbers. Timing and counting and quotas were everything. I figured out that if Jamie crept all day at his slowest rate, a mere ten yards a minute, then it would take almost six hours to creep two miles. If, on the other hand, he crept at his top speed of 40 yards a minute, he would creep two miles in just 1 ½ hours. As for crawling, if he moved his slowest, an unbearable five yards a minute, then it would take almost three hours to crawl the required ½ mile. And if he crawled as fast as he could all the time, which at the present was ten yards a minute, then he could finish in 1 ½ hours. I calculated further that 50 ladder walks took a little over an hour, 30 brachiates with help took a little less than an hour, 60 masks took exactly an hour, and patterning and reading together took a little less than an hour, for a total of four hours of program in addition to the creeping and crawling. Therefore, we would spend from a minimum of seven hours a day doing the program to a maximum of 13 hours a day.

On Day 8 I got Jamie to crawl 220 yards on the kitchen floor before school. That was one-fourth of his total crawling goal. Three things enabled him to do so much. For one thing, he woke up extra early, and I wasted no time in slipping on his elbow and knee pads. Secondly, Jennifer, to whom I had finally explained our expectations for her to do some creeping, crawling, and brachiating, crawled with him and provided competition. And thirdly, I devised a simple game that operated as an incentive. I challenged them at the end of each ten-yard lap around the table and back to the refrigerator to get another lap done before I could return to the kitchen from some errand. As they took off, I went down the hall and made a bed or put in a load of wash or changed Benjiman's diaper or got myself dressed or laid out their clothing or wiped toothpaste off the bathroom walls or organized the day's reading cards. I always made sure they beat me back to the refrigerator all 22 times. I got things done that needed to be done, while at the same time successfully supervising the program. The remainder of the program, conducted when Jamie was home from kindergarten, went so much smoother after having had such an early start.

On Day 15, I began to get Jamie up regularly at 5:30 a.m. He not only completed 220 yards of crawling before school from then on, but he also did ten ladder walks and 500 yards of creeping on the upstairs course. That was less than the 880 yards that was supposed to be done at once, but we had to do what amount fit in best in the time we had, and make up the rest later. Fear of missing the bus proved to be a fabulous incentive. More than once he was just coming down the hall to the living room, after having crept in and out of all the bedrooms and the bathrooms, when I yelled "Bus!" and he crept to the door at lightning speed, stood up, and ran out the door and down the short walkway to the beloved bus that would take him on a 3 ½ hour furlough from duty. On those days that we cut the timing so close, he went to school with his knee pads still on under his jeans.

I became a drill master. I barked out orders and expected full coopera-tion and immediate response with no questions asked. "Jamie, drop down and do 500 yards!" "Jamie, let's knock off five brachiates. Look, grab, squeeze. Look, grab, squeeze." "Hurry up or you won't get that ten-minute break this afternoon!" I wondered how other mothers, less organized and less driven than I, managed to conduct the program. Were there really others doing what I was doing? In contrast to Alden, who could calmly read a newspaper during a traffic jam, I always did everything according to a plan, and at a frenzied pace. I put away glasses in the cupboard with such haste that I often broke them, and I always ran up the stairs, being careful to step either to the extreme left or the extreme right of each carpeted step so as to prevent excess weight in the middle where everyone else stepped. I stood at the wastebasket to read my mail and threw it away immediately, even birthday cards. I read the headlines and weather in our daily newspa-per as soon as it came at 3 P.M. and then I threw it away. Alden knew just where to find it when he wanted to settle down with after supper. My jewelery box had to be at a precise angle on my bureau, and the kitchen chairs had to be lined up with a certain square on the linoleum. Thus I thought I really could make a good effort at the demands of the program assigned to us. In fact, I found I would do anything to try to reach the magic numbers the Institutes had given us. I tried seven days a week, through Mother's Day and my 33rd birthday. As Jamie was a slave to me, so I was a slave to the numbers. Twenty-nine brachiates would not do. He must reach 30. Only 1 ¾ miles of creeping was no good. The prescribed two miles was the acceptable amount. Even if it meant Jamie could no longer afford time out for sit-down meals. I fed him a spoonful at a time from a plate on the floor as he went by. When some scrambled egg tumbled out of his mouth onto the kitchen floor as he was crawling early in the morning, I yelled, "Keep your mouth closed! Jennifer doesn't want to crawl in egg!"

More than once I asked myself if my demands or threats constituted abuse or cruelty. Could my neighbors hear the yelling? Jamie was not always cooperative. I was neglecting two of my children to do this program, and the third one wished I would neglect him. What did the tone of my constant commands do to my image as a loving mother in the eyes of Jennifer and Benjiman, who cringed when they could not get out of earshot? What were my bizarre expectations doing to my relationship with Jamie? Would he eventually love me for it or would he hate me forever? Or did that depend on the outcome? He often turned and ran when he saw me coming. I would find him under his bed or under his covers or in the closet. One day when the pool was first opened and the water was still too icy cold for me, I let him go in for a quick swim. I couldn't get him out! He kept pushing off the edge just as I'd get close. He was blue and shivering—but to him that was better than the alternative of crawling. On other occasions he embarrassed me in front of volunteers. "It was still light out when we finished last night," or "Probably I can have a bite or two of my sandwich after this pattern."

It was impossible to explain to people not particularly close to us or not thoroughly informed on the Institutes' theories just what we were doing or why we were doing it. On Day 17, we went out to dinner with another couple. We kept talking about the program because that was what consumed our every minute, and they kept changing the subject, not understanding. They even asked us to take a week's vacation with them. We were in different worlds.

A few days later, Alden invited two other couples over for dinner, thinking that would be easier and less expensive than going out, and yet help us to feel like we were still part of the real world. Alden did the grocery shopping, cooking, and late evening cleaning up. I went to bed at midnight when our guests left and Alden finished the pots and pans at 2:00 a.m. For the first time he truly appreciated what I had always gone through when we had company.

In the morning, we decided it wasn't worth it. I was exhausted from several late nights of preparing word cards and filling in the tedious daily log that was required for the interim report to the Institutes. And my few hours of sleep were always interrupted by Benjimin and by the 5:30 alarm.

By Day 25, I was depressed. There was no way Jamie could creep two miles and crawl half a mile and brachiate 30 times all on the same day. The goals were ridiculously high and there was no time for normalcy. I feared I wasn't making the program "fun." What was fun about creeping and crawling and quotas? I still held onto my belief in the theory of it all, but the hours were questionable. Did it really matter exactly how much, as long as he was at it most of the time? Should I just cut everything in half and falsify the report? Did they assign parents too much on purpose as part of their whole psychological game—so that they would know that we were not really doing it if we didn't complain it was too much?

And why did we have to pay $250 a month when it was we who were doing all the work, 800 miles away from them? Our financial situation was approaching a crisis point. And our evenings were so busy cutting and marking word cards and filling out useless creeping and crawling logs that we barely had time to write out the check for the Institutes.

Jamie was becoming a zombie. His constant question was, "What number am I on?" I even heard him say it in his sleep one night. He lived for the five minutes he earned to put his pegs in his Lite-Brite toy or the ten minutes he earned to ride on his bicycle (with training wheels). He and I were both mechanical, robotlike. Sometimes, if I had inadvertently left the stop watch downstairs when I was upstairs, or inside when I was outside, I had to orally count off the seconds that Jamie had his mask on. And I counted right past 60, on up to 70 or 80 before I remembered what I was doing.

I became a midnight ice cream and chocolate sauce thief. Sometimes, when my longing was urgent or the time for making sauce short, I just grabbed a handful of chocolate bits and filled my mouth. I found that my capacity was 50, and often I methodically counted out another 50 while the first mouthful was slowly and deliciously melting in my cheek. Such sweets were, of course, taboo on the program, and the kids had no idea that I had ice cream hidden in the freezer or chocolate chips stashed in the cupboard. But it was the one thing I looked forward to every day. I tried to suppress the recurring thought as to what Jamie had to look forward to every day. Since I seldom went further than the mailbox, I had to indulge myself in some way. When I did get to go out on an errand, I wrote in my notebook, "I got out today," as if I were an escaped prisoner.

My sagging spirits received a much needed boost one day. First, as I showed Jamie a set of word cards in the morning, he said every word before I could say it! Later, Alden and I went to school for a conference with key school personnel concerning Jamie's progress and placement for the next fall. The principal, the guidance counselor, the nurse, the teacher, and the aide were there. Before the meeting, I chatted outside with Dixie Tarbell, his teacher. I had recently described to her Jamie's home program, and had loaned her Glenn Doman's book on brain injured children. Privately, she now confided to me that she thought the book was vital and that it really helped her understanding of the relationship of neurological development to learning. "It excited me, and believe me, I needed it at this point in my teaching," she said. She asked if she could come to see Jamie in action sometime.

Publicly, during the meeting, she described the encouraging observations she had made of Jamie in recent months: he spaced out less often, he needed less focusing from Lynne, the aide, his behavior was more goal oriented, he more often remembered what he was doing and finished it, he did not randomly move his head and eyes in space as before, he volunteered to read often, and he had greater confidence in and control of his body during recess and gym. She said she had reconsidered her previous position and now recommended that Jamie be promoted to first grade!

Just five days later, on Day 34, I came the rest of the way out of the doldrums. Jamie crept two miles and crawled half a mile for the first time! And on a school day! He met all his other goals, too. On other days I had given Jamie and Jennifer each one, two, three, or four nickels for their wallets, depending on the amount of program done. But this day deserved more than nickels. As soon as Jamie hit two miles, at 7:30 p.m., I got them into the car and headed for Dairy Queen. They couldn't believe their good fortune as they sat there licking their large chocolate dipped cones. Conspiratorially, we said, "Don't tell Glenn Doman!" They couldn't remember when they last had ice cream. And I couldn't remember when I had last had so much fun with them.

When we got home from DQ, Alden had two musician friends over for a jam session. I let Jamie join the group with his toy saxophone and Jennifer with her shakers. When I finally got Jamie into bed, I hoped he would have pleasant dreams.

I knew he might not repeat his performance again tomorrow, or even the next day, but at least now I knew that it could be done. It was not impossible. As soon as school was over for the summer, and we had those extra hours every day, it would be a cinch. We would meet all the goals every day, and have time for a swim or two besides. Maybe even some sit-down dinners. The only thing left to strive for before going back to Philadelphia was independent brachiation.

The last day of school was Friday, June 13, Day 44 of the program. I cried when I looked at his report card. At the bottom where it said what grade he would be in next fall, I could see where "K" had been erased and "1" inserted. Everything was going just fine now at home and at school. He was reading word cards and meeting physical goals, and he was going to first grade. The next day Alden brought me a dozen yellow roses and said, "Thank you for doing a good job with my son."

Now that school was out, we got more done earlier. Jamie was motivated by his own successes. He knew the goals and he became conscientious about reaching them. One night, as we were finishing a late supper at the table, I casually mentioned that he was only 500 yards short of creeping two miles, but that he needn't finish. He jumped up from the table and dropped down to his knees in the living room and began creeping the upstairs course. Another morning, he showed up in our bedroom before the 5:30 alarm all dressed and said, "Let's go!"

We usually stayed inside and worked like crazy until after lunch because he was less distracted and got more done inside. Surprisingly, he did most of his creeping around the patterning table in the therapy room.

He wasn't bored by repeating that short distance over and over. He seemed to enjoy hearing me click off lap after lap on the clicker so quickly, even though he had to do so many more laps to reach a specified distance than he would on the longer upstairs course. Choosing to creep around and around that table was to me like choosing to walk on a treadmill rather than along a scenic road.

As he crept around and around, sometimes I crept with him, sometimes Jennifer crept with him, sometimes I sat on the floor and gave him a "pep pill"—a raisin or a piece of dry cereal—as he went by, sometimes I challenged him to get around before I could say the alphabet, or sometimes I just told him stories about my youth at Spruce Mountain Lodge to keep his mind off what he was doing. One morning he reached one whole mile by 10:00, a few days later by 9:30, and a few days after that by 8:35!

I did all of Jamie's reading program indoors in the morning. Outside, the cards blew away, got dripped on, or had to compete with too interesting a background. Progress slowed considerably when he had to put up with watching neighbors playing on our gym set or Jennifer and a friend in the pool. One day there were thirteen kids in the pool! Jamie must have wondered why he was crawling and the rest of the world was playing.

In addition to enduring that sort of torture, he also got stung twice on his hand while creeping in the grass. He became understandably reluctant to creep outdoors after that, and on the rare occasions when he did creep outdoors along the pool fence, he slowed up considerably, looking for bees.

He got unbearably hot some days working outdoors. My solution for that was what became known as the "pickle dip." I held him by the wrists and lowered him into the pool, knee pads and all, and then pulled him right out and ushered him straight back to the crawl course, as this procedure was strictly for comfort, not pleasure. I too occasionally took a quick dip to cool off. We were always dressed in bathing suits.

I found along with cooling off our bodies on summer days, I also had to cool off the outdoor patterning table. I kept a towel soaked with pool water on it until just before using it. Otherwise the black vinyl was hot enough to fry the proverbial egg.

With the everpresent emphasis on numbers, Jamie's mastery of basic math concepts advanced beyond the simple addition and subtraction that we had seen him absorb during our initial efforts with him to beginning multiplication and division. I usually lined up nine rocks on the ground at the beginning of his outdoor crawling or creeping course. He pushed one away each time he finished a lap and that gave him a visual cue as to how much more he had left to do. But it also taught him what "nine" was made up of. After he had done three, and I asked him how many he had left to do, he was apt to say "Two threes." When creeping inside on the upstairs course, I usually lined up 18 raisins on the coffee table, one to be eaten after each lap. He soon learned that 18 was also divisible by three, and that he had three threes or four threes left to do. When he crept on the ten-yard circuit around the patterning table downstairs, or crawled on the ten-yard circuit in the kitchen, I always said he must do nine tens of creeping or two tens plus two of crawling, just because it sounded less staggering than to say that he must creep 90 times around that table or crawl 22 times around this table. But without planning to, I was teaching him the foundation of our number system. Tens and ones. Sometimes he would ask his favorite question, "What number am I on?" and I would pause in my storytelling to glance at the clicker that I was mechanically advancing each time he went by, and respond, "You are on the sixth one of your seventh ten," and he would say, "Oh, good, I only have 24 more to go." Such immediate and confident answers demonstrated to me an indisputable understanding of numbers.

Alden felt that Jamie's mind was becoming better organized in other ways too. He observed that he no longer laid on the floor pushing a truck and drooling all day. Instead, in the few short breaks Jamie was allowed every day, he did 100-piece puzzles unassisted, he created his own designs on his Lite Brite toy, he practiced on his two-wheeler or on his gym set or on his swimming, he carried on more intelligent conversations, and he remembered stories that he was told. We also considered it a sign of increased awareness that Jamie could not be coerced to do one yard more of creeping or crawling than his assigned goals were. He knew when he had reached two miles and that was as far as he would go. What incentive was there to hurry if in the end he would only have to do more instead of enjoying a well-deserved break? We, who also needed a break, endorsed Jamie's point of view wholeheartedly.

Alden also exclaimed over Jamie's improved physical condition from his daily workout. He measured his chest and was amazed to find that it was one inch bigger around already. His muscle tone was better too. Alden was even more enthused about Jamie's physical condition because Jamie seemed suddenly to be close to brachiating alone!

On Day 57, Alden started getting up at 5:30 a.m. with Jamie and me. He wanted to do a more fair share of the program with Jamie and to diminish my responsibilities a little. After I dressed Jamie in the clothes I had laid out the night before, fed him his vitamins and the first installment of his breakfast, usually fruit, masked him three times, and showed him three sets of word cards, he and Alden went downstairs to work together for one hour and 15 minutes. During that time I made sandwiches for lunch, retired old word cards and got out the new category, wrote in my journal, cooked eggs for Jamie's breakfast (at least 15 grams of protein was to be consumed in the morning), went downstairs to flash cards at Jamie, nursed Benjiman, and otherwise prepared myself for the day so that I would be less frantic later when I was alone with all three children. At first Alden did only a few ladder walks with Jamie and no creeping. I felt like we were losing ground and that I ought to take over. But I left them alone. Alden became more efficient—as I had learned to do in the beginning.

By the end of June, Jamie's schedule looked like this.

5:30-6	dressed, 3 masks, juice, fruit, vitamins, 3 sets of word cards
6-7:15	25 ladder walks and 500 yards of creeping with Daddy
7:15-7:45	crawl 220 yards in kitchen while being fed eggs
7:45-8	10 ladder walks
8-8:40	400 yards creeping upstairs
8:40-9	15 ladder walks
9-10	3 patterns, 900 yards creeping, 5 brachiates
10-10:15	break and snack
10:15-12	220 yards crawling in kitchen, 900 yards creeping upstairs, 5 brachiates, swim break before noon volunteers if time
12-1	3 patterns, 225 yards crawling outside, 5 brachiates
1-2	lunch and swim break
2-4:15	15 brachiates, 900 yards creeping outdoors
4:15-5	2 patterns, 220 yards crawling in kitchen

Masking every 7 minutes all day, except when creeping or crawling, until 80 done. Reading cards every few minutes in a.m. until done. Sometimes given choice of creeping or crawling in a time slot. On slow days, completed any unfinished crawling or creeping or brachiating or ladder walks after 5:00.

Dick was involved with the program on weekends. Susan usually was too but at this particular time she was away on a five-week train trip across Canada with friends. Dick came to our house faithfully every Saturday morning. He did more than just pattern. He held Jamie while he tried to brachiate, and he walked back and forth beside Jamie as he crawled on the outdoor course. Once I heard him say to Jamie, as he held out a sandwich for Jamie to take a bite from as he crawled by, that if he could crawl and eat lunch at the same time, then he could be President some day. Dick also patiently told Jamie story after story as he walked along beside him those hot summer afternoons. Some stories were fabricated, usually about Superman, and some were factual, of which Jamie had a favorite, the story of the Titanic.

Dick was always thinking of ways to help Jamie. Even before we went on the program, he once designed a simple splint of metal and tape to keep Jamie's hand open, and another time he drew plans for a system of weights and pulleys to strengthen Jamie's grip and muscles. Still another time, he brought with him a small rectangular sponge for Jamie to practice holding and squeezing with his right hand.

But Dick's most ingenious contribution to Jamie's welfare was a contraption he made to help Jamie brachiate. It had all kinds of straps and little wheels that rolled along the two boards on each side of the rungs. Once in it, Jamie could go for a roller coaster ride! Though we appreciated the thought and the effort, we immediately disapproved, partly because it was awkward and it took time to get into but mostly because it gave constant support and therefore deviated too much from the ultimate goal of independent brachiation.

Many of our other volunteers were equally remarkable in their dedication to us. Anita came twice a week and stayed for hours. She measured and cut cardboard for me, washed out grungy masks and readied new ones for use, took Benjiman for strolls, read to Jennifer or took her for a ride in her car, did errands for me, brought some pieces of foam to make inexpensive knee pads for my own sore knees, brought Jamie and Jennifer unexpected toys and treats, brought along a friend to pattern if her regular partner couldn't make it, vacuumed the pool, and became a closer friend. She often made lunch for us all and then brought it out to where Jamie and Jennifer were creeping or crawling around the pool area. She also made frequent trips into the house for juice mixed with powered vitamin C, or for diaper changes.

Judi, another ever present volunteer, brought us countless lunches and suppers, and always took Jennifer home with her for the afternoon after her hour of patterning. Susan Monday came the shortest distance but with the most difficulty because of the many children she took care of. She came at 8:00 a.m. on Saturday mornings before Susan and Dick arrived, and she came numerous other times at a moment's notice—in the middle of lunch for ten kids or in the middle of a thunderstorm. Jane was another gem. She was the most vivacious and hip-looking grandmother I had ever seen. She happened to live near the store that had the cheapest poster board and she picked up piles of it for me, and then turned it into 9" x 3" blank cards for me when she got home. Cora Jo was always looking out for Benjiman's safety. She was appalled when I laid him and his blanket on the bricks under the picnic table (shade was scarce out there), or when he was all slouched up in his automatic swing (it kept him quiet, though), or when I laid him near the raised hearth in the TV room (because of her I had to purchase a thick rug that went up over the bricks).

Cora Jo also provided me with a source of much-needed volunteers— her neighbor's church group. That neighbor was Darlene. Besides arranging for several of her group to come at needed times, Darlene herself probably was my most dependable volunteer. She never canceled, came extra times to substitute, shortened my bathrobe for me, and her daughters substituted on a long-term basis when someone went on vacation. Once she told the school nurse, who called her at home one morning to say she should pick up her daughter immediately because her arm was inexplicably numb, that she would be right there to get her daughter but the trip to the emergency room would have to be delayed an hour as she was just on her way out the door to pattern!

The list of one-time patterners was long. We frequently engaged the services of anyone who was passing through. My father, Alden's cousin, Susan's niece, sister, and mother, Marj's mother and sister, Piera's husband, Jane's daughter, one of my college roommates who was visiting for the day and brought supper with her for her family and mine, a childhood chum who happened to drop in, and a total stranger, who was attending a two-day seminar on natural foods with Susan Monday and who, having no other place to stay, had spent the night sleeping under her willow tree! I often wondered what went though the heads of those who were involved so briefly. Did they think we were insane? How could they understand?

Dixie Tarbell, Jamie's kindergarten teacher, came to observe one day at the beginning of July. It was Day 64. She was so interested that I assigned her a regular patterning spot. Pattianne frequently didn't show up for one of her two times, so I called her to say I had another person and would now only need her once a week, hoping that that way she would be more reliable. Jamie was thrilled to have his teacher coming every week to help him. After only a few visits, I could see that Dixie was really absorbed by the program. She confided to me that she was trying to organize the different levels of her brain by creeping a little every day, indoors and outside in her garden, and that she increased the oxygen supply to her brain by using sandwich bags to mask herself.

Though I no longer had the time to curl my hair or polish my nails, the one thing I did not give up was reading my issue of *Time* magazine each week. I had been compulsive about that for ten years and I wasn't going to stop now. Just when doubts about the program were again creeping into the forefront of my consciousness, Time did a cover story on backache in the July 7 issue. It stated that the cause of back pain is man's upright posture. We should have stayed in the creep position, it said! And some patients reported they got relief by hanging! Though Jamie's chief symptom was not backache, the remedies suggested in this article at least made me feel that the Institutes' program might not be as totally irrational as I sometimes imagined.

Jennifer was becoming sassy and rebellious. It was exceedingly difficult to get her to do any program. She either sneaked away out of my sight before I could tell her to creep or crawl or brachiate, or she outright defied my instructions. Perhaps it was because she sensed that my main intentions were with Jamie and that she was just an experiment on the side. It was true that I was often inconsistent in my requirements of her and that I drove Jamie harder. Or perhaps her defiance came out simply because she had a stronger personality than Jamie and dared to disobey me. At the beginning, she had thought of it all as a sort of game. She enjoyed competition and she was unusually perceptive of her brother's needs. She had whispered to me one day, "Mom, when I go speedy, Jamie goes speedy!" But she was no longer the motivator she had once been. She cheated and lied about how many laps she had done, and she fought constantly with Jamie about who had the most done. Other times she followed me around saying, "I love you, Mom, I love you," as if trying to convince herself.

And then she developed an alarming habit. She began urinating everywhere but in the bathroom. She went on the thick green shag carpet in her room, on our downhill driveway, on the cement cellar floor, on the rug under the brachiating ladder, and on one of Jamie's favorite puzzles.

Our first step toward rectifying the situation was to take Jennifer off the program. We had seen no change in her crossed eye, and it was by far more important to preserve her sanity and to reestablish her positive relationship with me than pursuing a questionable hope of throwing away her glasses. I didn't make any big deal about it. I didn't want them to think that we ever even remotely questioned the value of the program. I just said that it was too hard for me to keep track in my notebook of what she had done too, and that we would just let her pretty glasses do the job of uncrossing her eye. On Monday, July 21, Day 82 for us, Day 261 for the Iranian hostages, Jennifer was set free.

As the time neared for us to return to Philadelphia, I sank into another depression. Except for independent brachiation, which I still saw as an impossibility, Jamie was meeting his goals. But what difference had that made, and what kind of a life was it for any of us? I tried to make it fun, but it just wasn't the sort of thing that most people enjoyed. It was grueling and repetitious. Evenings were gobbled up making word cards and keeping the log. I was exhausted all the time. I fell asleep on the living room floor three Saturday nights in a row while trying to entertain Dick and other visitors. One Sunday afternoon I fell asleep on the patterning table during a break. When I sat on the floor to encourage Jamie to new rates of speed in crawling and creeping, I nodded off.

We tried to do things that a normal family enjoys in the summertime. We took the kids out for pizza and then to the movie theatre to see *The Black Stallion*, and we all fell asleep. We took them to Prescott Park to hear live music and to see a play, and we all fell asleep. Alden and I went to the Hampton Casino to listen to Maria Muldaur. They asked for my ID at the door and since I was more than a dozen years over the drinking age, my elation at having been asked kept me awake for a while. But Maria Muldaur didn't come on stage until 11:00, and then, even as loud as the music was, we couldn't keep our eyes open. We left before midnight.

No fireworks on the Fourth. No celebration on our eighth anniversary.

Only one short sail on Dick's boat—and that in a thunderstorm. I seldom swam in our pool, and I never sunbathed. I had only taken Benjiman in the water a few times. Though I had gotten him to the point where he didn't mind being ducked under water, I wished that I could have more time with him in the pool. My life was so dull that the tiniest deviation brought me great excitement. Like the morning I cracked three eggs in a row and all three were double yolks. For days I told everyone I saw about it.

Benjiman was growing and changing before I had a chance to notice. He hitched forward easily when left on the crawl course or on the kitchen floor. Had it not been for my training at the Institutes, I would surely have left him in his infant seat all day and he wouldn't have moved on his own so soon. He had also lately been getting up onto his knees—the "quad position" the Institutes called it—in preparation for creeping.

I started feeding Benjiman some cereal because he was waking more frequently in the night, and I felt he needed more than just milk, especially with his increased mobility. But on the other hand, for five months I had revelled in the fact that his every fingernail and hair grew because of me. Now that bond was forever broken and I missed it. One of the volunteers usually fed him his morning cereal while I worked with Jamie. And when I did nurse Benjiman, it was seldom a quiet or private experience. I was always walking around with him attached—following Jamie as he crept or getting out juice and a snack or slipping on a mask. There was no time to sit still. When I nursed Jennifer I had always put my other arm around Jamie and read a story to him. But now I was always in a hurry. Jamie, like his little brother, was also used to eating on the run. Alden took a photograph of the typical mealtime in our house. It showed me feeding both my sons at once. I was sitting in a chair, nursing Benjiman, with my feet up on the patterning table to make a tunnel for Jamie to creep through. I had a plate on my lap, balanced beside Benjiman, and was feeding Jamie a mouthful as he emerged from the tunnel.

Jennifer, too, was growing away from me. I saw so little of her as volunteers read to her or she entertained herself or Judi took her home with her. And she was still urinating on the floor.

Susan, on whom I depended for moral support almost as much as I did on Alden, was away. Not only did I miss her, but I was acutely aware that while she leisurely looked at the magnificent Rockies every day and ate gourmet meals at a different restaurant every night, I was locked into a dull and unrewarding routine.

Jamie's left shoulder ached constantly and both of his hands were blistered and bleeding all over again as in the beginning because I was giving him less support and he was having to work harder when trying to brachiate. He cried every day and said he hated to brachiate. Should I push him harder despite the pain or should I give up trying to reach the impossible? I was not only unsure that I was administering the program properly to Jamie, but what about Benjiman and Jennifer? I hadn't made any word cards for Benjiman, as had been recommended. Should I have? I no longer required Jennifer to crawl, creep, or brachiate when I had been told that such measures would positively uncross her eye. How had I dared to have her stop? Was I failing all three of my children?

I had one more worry on my mind. In the lengthy and time-consuming interim report to the Institutes, we had mentioned that Jamie had improved in school so much that he was considered capable of handling first grade. A week later I got back a crisp note from our advocate that said:

Dear Mr. and Mrs. Bratt:

There is one point I must make crystal clear. Jamieson cannot go to school and be on the Institutes' program at the same time. This is policy. It is our job to get Jamieson well as quickly as possible. If you have time to do the full program and send him to school, you should be using his extra time by doing extra program. He'll get well that much quicker and be able to go to school full time sooner. Please inform me in writing what you decide.

I couldn't decide.

18
Lucky to be Brain Injured

Stop the pity and the pennies. Stop the millions that go for adjusting the child to his "afflictions," that go for programs to help him "live with his difficulties." Go take a new look at these children. Then—help them to get well.

Napear, 1974, p. 428

Wednesday, July 23, had been different from the start. I hadn't had to say, "Look, grab, squeeze" all day to Jamie because he was looking, grabbing, and squeezing all on his own. There was new determination in his eyes, and the wooden rungs creaked under the intensity of his grip. The fingers on his right hand stayed closed around the rungs long enough for his left hand to let go and reach for the next rung. Almost imperceptibly, I began to lessen my support. Neither of us spoke all day of what was happening for fear of bursting the bubble. It happened during the late afternoon, when we were almost done with everything. We were out by the pool, and I was trying to get up the courage to let go of him completely. I did in in the middle of brachiate number 24. Jamie brachiated all alone for four rungs, before dropping to the ground.

After we stopped jumping up and down, we went straight to Dairy Queen, saying, "Don't tell Glenn Doman!" all the way. My jubilance surpassed what I had felt when he had first crept two miles and crawled half a mile. This was to me infinitely more important. It meant he could use his right hand if he tried hard enough. My fantasies of completely curing Jamie and of taking him around to all his former doctors to show him off came rushing back to me. Long ago I had promised to take them to an amusement park at the beach if Jamie ever went all the way across the ladder alone. I knew now that we would go.

That night Alden and I made the decision to keep Jamie out of school in the fall and to continue full time with whatever the Institues wanted us to do.

Two days later, Alden and I drove both cars to Portland in the evening to pick up Susan and her friends who were arriving back in the States on a ferry from Canada. We couldn't wait to tell her about the breakthrough. Jamie had on his green T-shirt that said "I'M A LITTLE CREEP" on the front and "I CREEP TWO MILES A DAY" on the back. People stared at his shirt questioningly as he raced around the dock, watching anxiously for the big white ship to come into view. It didn't bother me that they stared—I felt comfortable and secure with what we were doing for him.

Soon Susan was embracing her three favorite kids and loading her suitcases into our car. Everyone spent the night with us, and then the other couple and their three children went home with a friend who came for them the next morning. Susan got a ride home with Dick Sunday night, after spending the weekend with us, recounting her journey, and rejoicing over the new hope for Jamie.

The original revisit to the Institutes for our whole group had been scheduled for this week, but was postponed for two weeks because Glenn Doman had to speak to the annual convention of the United Mine Workers Union. They contribute a certain amount of financial support to the Institutes each year, and all they ask in return is that Glenn Doman present to them the case history of a child who has achieved success on the program. I dreamed that some day Jamie would be the one presented at this gathering.

There were only two weeks left until we returned to Philadelphia. Could Jamie brachiate the full length of the ladder before then? In addition to the ultimate incentive of the amusement park, I told him that I would take him to Dunkin' Donuts when he carried himself for six rungs, and out to dinner when he did ten rungs. First thing Monday morning he did six rungs, and we went to Dunkin' Donuts after the 9:00 patterners left. Jamie had a powdered sugar donut and Jennifer had a chocolate frosted one and Benjiman tried to drink some juice out of a glass. As the forbidden sugar was consumed, we said again, "Don't tell Glenn Doman!"

Independent brachiation was excruciatingly strenuous business. I myself could not go all the way across the ladder, but then I hadn't conditioned myself to do it for five months as had Jamie. Still, it was like pulling teeth to get him to go just one or two rungs alone a day. His mood and determination had to be just right. I spouted off to all the volunteers and other friends who came that he could do some alone. But they never witnessed it. They only observed me supporting him under the ladder as usual, and probably thought that I was having delusions. "Poor girl, she finally went over the edge," their eyes said. I eliminated most of the ladder walks because they seemed useless, and we needed the extra time for brachiating. Each trip across the 12-foot ladder took longer now that I was barely holding him.

On Sunday, August 4, Day 95, I went to a baby shower in the afternoon. Alden surprised me by telling me that morning that he and Dick would supervise Jamie all day—not just while I was gone in the afternoon. I had the day off! I only appeared for patterning and to flash reading cards. It was heaven. No pressure and no counting. When I arrived at the shower, I was totally relaxed and rejuvenated. I was the last one to leave the party. When I finally got home, I had the biggest surprise of all awaiting me. Jamie had brachiated the entire length of the ladder alone!

Dick had coerced him by telling him that he would go as many rungs as Jamie did—not really expecting that he would have to go more than one or two. Though I missed Jamie's feat by a few minutes, I arrived home just in time to see Dick brachiate across the ladder. He moaned in genuine agony as he forced his unfit body to fulfill his promise, while Jamie doubled over in laughter.

We chose Wednesday afternoon to go to the amusement park at Salisbury Beach because it was Kiddies' Day and all rides were half price. Jamie worked his hardest and fastest ever in eager anticipation of quitting time. He pushed hard and took no breaks. He crawled half a mile in only 60 minutes, and he crept two miles in only 145 minutes. He previously had averaged about 112 minutes and 223 minutes. He did no independent brachiates, though he worked at it. Daddy came home at 3:00 and I had already canceled the late afternoon patterner. It had been cloudy all day and by 3:00 it was sprinkling. But we had no intention of delaying the celebration another minute. The rain was light and intermittent and did not at all interfere with our pleasure. Jamie and Jennifer went on the merry-go-round, the little boats, the little cars, the little airplanes, in the haunted house, and on the ferris wheel with me in between them. They ate junk food from every vendor we passed. Jennifer got pink cotton candy all over her glasses. "Don't tell Glenn Doman" was the standard refrain at every stop. Benjiman sat in his stroller in the midst of all the noise and commotion and looked shell-shocked. Many hours later, we put three exhausted but happy children to bed, and Alden and I finished up the celebration with a refreshing skinny dip.

Saturday, August 9, was the last day before we were to leave for Philadelphia to find out what our new program would be. We had done the old program for 101 days. Alden and I took stock of Jamie's achievements. He crept and crawled long distances every day with increasing speed, agility, and willingness. He used his right arm swimming and could now keep his head above the water. He held onto his bicycle handlebar longer and he pumped his legs when swinging. He had brachiated the full length of the ladder alone. Though he had thus far been unable to repeat that momentous accomplishment, we knew that he would do it regularly soon.

Jamie had also learned to read in those 101 days. It had happened so gradually that it didn't get the attention that independent brachiation had. But he had definitely crossed the line. He was a reader. He read simple books on his own, and he learned new words easily. More importantly, he enjoyed reading. I had done something extra, beyond the flash cards, and I felt that it had made the difference. In June I had started taping blank sheets of paper to the wall and several times a day I had written out a few sentences as I spoke them. Jamie watched and listened.

"I went out to the garden. I got lots of lettuce. We will make a salad."
"Daddy is home. I can hear him upstairs. What did he bring for supper?"
"Jamie got hurt today. There was a little blood. Mommy cleaned it. It will
be all be better soon." "We will brachiate and creep before the next cross
pattern. Anita will be here in 30 minutes. We will look at the clock. The
second hand moves fast. The minute hand moves slowly." "Uncle Dick
slept on the top bunk last night. When Jamie gets bigger, he will sleep on the
top bunk and Benji will sleep on the bottom bunk. Then where will Dick
sleep?"

This method made more sense to me than single words flashed at high
speed. It flowed and it was entertaining. As sheets got filled up, I moved
them up toward the ceiling and taped fresh blank sheets down low at
Jamie's eye level. The whole therapy room was covered with our new
wallpaper. By August, Jamie was reading the words out loud to me as I
silently wrote them.

We had many reasons to be proud of Jamie. We had many reasons to
return to the Institutes. Glenn Doman had said that because of the intense
attention given to a brain injured child on the program, most brain injured
children, whom many had formerly thought to be slow, turned out brighter
than normal children. We could now see that potential.

"We are lucky that he is brain injured," we said.

19

I'm Gonna Win!

Scientists in Philadelphia are not only saving hundreds of mentally crippled children from lives of blackout and isolation but are actually teaching many of them to outperform their normal brothers and sisters.

Beck, September 12, 1964, p. 26

This time we were not leaving Jennifer behind. She had finally stopped urinating around the house, and we didn't want her to have a relapse. Besides, the Institutes, we now knew, was an informal place where we would meet old friends, and Jennifer would be perfectly welcome.

This time we would be staying with my sister Guilene. Her apartment was only a, half hour away from the Institutes, and as we expected our schedule to be less rigorous this time, that was not an unreasonable distance. The kids would have to sleep on the floor, but at least there would be no bill to pay at the end of the week.

We dreaded the long drive to Philadelphia in the August heat. We would be even more crowded than the last time because Susan was going again and there was an extra child. Jamie and Jennifer would take turns sitting on either Susan's or my lap. That meant that one child would always be loose, not buckled safely in a seat belt. I didn't like that, but we had no choice. Benjiman, now almost six months old, would probably sleep most of the way, as he had before. Susan was tempted to fly down and meet us there, but she bravely decided to endure it with the Bratts.

The ride was remarkably comfortable and peaceful. We fed the kids and ourselves a steady supply of juice and snacks, and Susan and I sang songs and played games until we were exhausted. We pulled into my sister's parking lot at 5:00 p.m., and hit every one of the newly laid speed bumps with our overloaded, low-riding car as we made our way to her building. Laden with suitcases, diaper boxes, and sleeping bags, we knocked on Guilene's door.

We had dinner and a pleasant evening together, and then woke up Monday morning refreshed and anxious to tell the Institutes about Jamie's improvements that had taken place since we had sent them our mid-term report. He had brachiated alone all the way across the ladder and he could read. We were positively bubbly about it.

In the large, familiar waiting room, we greeted families and children we had become especially friendly with before. We noticed, as we looked around the room, that there were many more families missing from our original group than the one that Glenn Doman had predicted would not return.

We had four short appointments that morning: revisit history, physical measurements (height, weight, and chest), respiratory measurements, and a neurological assessment. After lunch, we had two brief meetings with different people explaining the results of the reevaluation, and a summary of his progress. They were pleased with Jamie's accomplishments. Glenn Doman's son, wearing a black blazer representing the Institute for the Achievement of Physical Excellence, told us that it was unusual to reach independent brachiation in the first three months. He told us of a little girl whose family had worked three years with her before she brachiated alone. She was now completely cured, but it had been a long haul. For us, it would be sooner.

We were done very early and went back to Guilene's for a swim in the complex's outdoor pool. There were a few residents relaxing quietly in the sun, and they looked up nervously through their sunglasses when they heard strangers with three little children approaching. As soon as they realized that we were not obnoxious company, they sank back into their lounge chairs and enjoyed watching the competence of my six-year-old and my four-year-old in the water and on the diving board. I particularly relished their shocked looks when I went underwater with an uncomplaining Benjiman several times.

The next two days we were to spend attending lectures by Glenn Doman and his senior staff members in the cold auditorium. Again they were very gracious about taking care of Benjiman and Jennifer along with Jamie in the waiting room, where they would be observing the children on the program and deciding on program changes. Again they would bring Benjiman to me when he needed to be fed, though it would be less often this time as he was older and taking some solid foods. We were the only family with two extra children along, as well as an extra adult.

After we dropped off our three children on Tuesday morning, we went to the lobby of the auditorium to socialize with other parents. Most were still enthused about the program or they would not have returned, but none had as much success as we felt we had experienced. At the sound of the bells, everyone quickly took an assigned seat and waited expectantly.

The first order of the day was to publicly congratulate the parents of those children who had made the most progress in various areas. A lady in a black blazer, Physical Excellence, and a lady in a tan blazer, Intellectual Excellence, stood at each of the two lecterns. There were several categories of achievement, and as a child's name was read and his or her achievement announced, the group responded with a round of applause. One child had crept for the first time, another had responded to a sound for the first time. Jamie, to our surprise, received three rounds of applause—for completing daily the most strenuous program for his age, for having been shown the most new words, and for having exceeded the requirements of the reading program. Everyone's eyes were on us. I blinked back proud tears.

Finally, Glenn Doman strode onto the stage. After welcoming us and congratulating us, he began an explanation of a brand new and revolutionary technique of monumental importance to brain injured children. It was called respiratory patterning. It was somewhat dangerous because it dealt with a vital function—breathing, and therefore was not taught to newcomers, but only to families who had proven themselves committed to the program and able to follow instructions explicitly.

A world famous anthropologist, Professor Raymond Dart, who was now semi-retired at age 87, and who worked closely with the Institutes for the Achievement of Human Potential, had noticed some time ago that brain injured children do not breathe properly. And no human being can do anything else perfectly unless he is first breathing smoothly, effortlessly, rhythmically, and automatically. A very hurt child cannot do anything because all of his concentration is centered on just breathing. A mildly hurt child cannot do anything normally because so much of his concentration is centered on breathing. For example, witness the long distance runner who collapses at the finish line, said Glenn Doman. He doesn't want to do anything but get his breath back. He is, for the moment, like a brain injured person. The only difference is that he will recover in a few minutes. The collapsed runner will go from being severely brain injured to moderately brain injured to mildly brain injured to normal. Brain injured children stay the way they are, poor breathers, all the time.

At this point, Glenn Doman staged a realistic demonstration of what happens to a normal person's ability to perform a task when his breathing is stressed. He asked for two volunteers. He had the female volunteer sing a song and the male volunteer read a paragraph. Then he told them to run around and around the lecture hall as many times as they could. They had to go up many steps on one side and down many steps on the other side. After many circuits, Glenn Doman stopped the two runners, and asked them to repeat their tasks. The woman could not sing and the man could not read. Mr. Doman had made his point.

The solution to this problem of poor breathing by brain injured children, who will not regain their abilities in just a few minutes, is to pattern the brain, to teach the injured brain how it feels to breathe properly so that the brain will eventually take over on its own. Then the child can put more effort into sensory reception. And once that has improved, his motor output might also improve.

Glenn Doman then pointed out a case where respiratory patterning had actually worked. Everyone had heard of Karen Ann Quinlan, the young girl who had been in a coma for years after mixing alcohol and drugs. The first time that her doctors turned off the respirator just to see what would happen, she stopped breathing, and the doctors quickly reconnected the respirator. Some time later, the family decided to disconnect the respirator, this time permanently, no matter what happened. To everyone's surprise, Karen Ann Quinlan continued to breathe on her own. She did not die.

But Glenn Doman and Professor Dart were not surprised by her survival. They alone knew the explanation. The respirator had patterned her brain. At the time of the first turn off, the brain had not been patterned with enough frequency, intensity, or duration. Later, at the time of the second turn off, Karen Ann Quinlan's brain had been sufficiently patterned to breathe on its own!

This information gave Glenn Doman's theory of respiratory patterning a great deal of credibility with the parents in the auditorium. He even hinted that greater progress could be made in the Quinlan case, but no one had asked him.

A little girl was brought in, and two staff members put a cloth respiratory vest on her chest and sat on opposite sides of her, and rhythmically pulled and released on long straps coming off the vest. In so doing they alternately compressed and released her chest in a prescribed way. We would all be individually instructed in the art of respiratory patterning on our own children at the end of the week.

During the hourly ten-minute breaks, we all talked eagerly about this new patterning. It would bring about miracles, we were all convinced. No matter what his middle initial was or was not, what a genius was this Glenn Doman! I had indeed noticed that Jamie seemed to hold his breath for no apparent reason, followed by a big gulp of air a few seconds later. Now I knew that it was important to change this, and that we could change this, and I could hardly wait to start. Buoyed by our three rounds of applause and by the hope offered by respiratory patterning. I bought Jamie a T-shirt that had an imprint of the Institutes' logo, a silhouetted figure walking off a large hand, and the words "I'M GONNA WIN!"

There were two more topics covered in that day's lectures. Just before lunch, there was an hour devoted to nutrition. The goals of the Institute for Physiological Excellence were reiterated: abundant health, superb function, robust structure. A lady in a maroon blazer explained that all we consume may be divided into three categories—food, vitamins, and minerals. This lecture would be concerned with food. Vitamins would be discussed at the next revisit, minerals at the revisit after that. She then talked at length about each of the categories of food—proteins, fats, and carbohydrates, with extra special attention paid to demon sugar.

After lunch, we were introduced to another new technique—new to us, that is, but not new at the Institutes. The vestibular growth program, said Glenn Doman's son with conviction, is a natural part of the program, yet is also the most deceptive part of the program. It looks like torture to an outsider. In reality, hurt and well kids alike love it. Babies love to be rocked and older kids love amusement park rides. So our reward for Jamie's first independent brachiation had not been a forbidden treat after all, I thought as I took notes.

Vestibular stimulation means putting a body in every position possible in relation to gravity and then moving the body through every plane and axis possible at three intensities—fast, slow, and start and stop. Negative newspaper accounts love to describe how kids on the Institutes' program are hung upside down and spun around, we were told. But they don't understand why it is being done or that the kids enjoy it so much.

Three components could be observed in movement, young Mr. Doman told us—coordination, breathing, and balance. The Institutes improve a brain injured child's coordination by cross patterning him. The Institutes improve a brain injured child's breathing by respiratory patterning. And the Institutes improve a brain injured child's balance by the vestibular program. The vestibular mechanism, which controls balance and orientation, is found in the ears and in the cerebellum. Stimulation not only enhances the balance and orientation vital to perfect movement, but it also physically "grows the brain." And brain growth is vital because new parts of the brain are needed to learn what injured parts of the brain no longer know.

That is the very foundation of Glenn Doman's whole theory. We must constantly send messages to the brain—in the form of visual, auditory, and tactile stimulation of increased frequency, intensity, and duration. And we must "grow the brain" to receive these messages. That vestibular stimulation does in fact grow the brain had been proven in recent research. Pups reared in a revolving environment had vestibular mechanisms in their brains 22-35% larger than pups reared in a normal environment.

There are two types of vestibular stimulation—passive, where someone does it to the child and the child has only to soak it up, and active, where the child does it to himself. Nine variations of passive vestibular stimulation were described. For example, horizontal rotation, head out, means the child is placed on some sort of support horizontal to the floor and, with the feet at the center of an imaginary circle, the whole body is rotated in a circular motion, with the head drawing an imaginary circumference horizontal to the floor. Vertical pirouetting, head down, means the child is placed upside down and spun around on a vertical axis parallel to the spine. T•/enty-nine active vestibular activities were also suggested, from somersaulting to jumping rope to swinging.

The lectures for the day were concluded with a practicum. From now on, at each revisit there would be a practicum for the parents. We were each given a pair of coveralls and asked to come down to the stage one row at a time to crawl across from one side to the other. It was quite comical because many parents really could not do it. We were told that that was because our big powerful cortex was trying to control the movement. We were trying to think about it, and it came out sloppy. Therefore, don't tell your kid how to do it. Just let him do it and talk about something else. He will eventually do it perfectly because the lower levels of the brain were being patterned to do it perfectly. The lessons were over by midafternoon and we were free to pick up our children and go sightseeing or whatever. We chose to go sightseeing.

As we gazed at the Liberty Bell, I found my thoughts wandering to respiratory patterning and vestibular stimulation. Frightening images of controlling Jamie's breathing and spinning him about like a top kept breaking into my mind. We had convinced friends, relatives, and volunteers of the validity of creeping and crawling and brachiating and cross patterning. But would I be able to successfully convey to others the necessity for these bizarre new techniques? I pictured myself chatting casually with my volunteers, who would be sitting on the redwood furniture by the pool between patternings, drinking the iced tea I had prepared for them, as I nonchalantly gave Jamie, who would be hanging upside down from the ladder, another mighty twirl.

The next day, Wednesday, Glenn Doman talked to the parents about intelligence. He prefaced his presentation with the assurance that this subject is by far the most exciting and most important of all. Intelligence tests are nonsense, he said. Intelligence is something that people recognize but can't define. We all know among our friends who is the brightest and who is the dullest. The world accepts and forgives paralysis, said Doman, but the world does not accept or forgive lack of intelligence. But that does not matter because it is a hundred times easier to make a child smart than it is to make him walk!

Every child has a higher potential intelligence than Leonardo da Vinci ever used. Doman said this three times, as was his habit, to make sure we internalized it. All we have to do is provide a stimulating environment and a steady diet of useful facts. Geniuses are made, not born. The only time the Institutes could not make a child bright is if the mother is convinced that the kid is an idiot. Mothers are the best teachers, and the mother and her child are the best learning team possible. The key in the learning situation is success. If you want a kid to learn, all you have to do is arrange for him to win. Unfortunately, our whole school system, said Glenn Doman with disgust, is set up to make children aware of their failures and not their successes. One wrong on the spelling test and there is a big red "X" at the top of the page. Motivation springs from success, not vice versa. We all do the things we do well over and over, and avoid the things that we know we don't do well.

Tiny children would rather learn than eat, said Glenn Doman with enthusiasm. Though formal education tragically does not begin until age six, learning actually begins at birth, or before. Games and toys have been created by adults too busy to talk to their children. Tiny children one year old or less would rather learn a complicated foreign language than play peek-a-boo or stare at a toy car. A one-year-old can be taught anything, from reading to math, more easily than a seven-year-old can be taught the same thing, as long as it is presented in an organized, clear, and factual manner. It is easy to make a tiny baby a genius, said Glenn Doman.

We would begin to make our hurt children into geniuses by using the Bits of Intelligence program. Glenn Doman had given us the background for this part of the program, and he now left the room while another staff member explained the mechanics of it.

Bits of intelligence are pictures mounted on poster board and grouped by categories. The pictures must be discrete—one item only, precise—accurate photos or drawings only, nonambiguous—labeled "black capped chickadee," not just "bird." It must be new to the child, otherwise intelligence will not be increased. Suitable pictures could be found in magazines, especially in wildlife magazines, on posters, on museum cards, in books. We were given a list of suggested categories, from national flags to famous sculptures to portraits of first ladies. We were also given a list of places to write for posters, magazine subscriptions, booklets, prints, and cards. Now we knew why we were subscribing to Ranger Rick and Safari Cards.

Any distracting background should be cut out of all pictures used, and then the picture should be mounted on an 11 x 11 inch piece of poster board. The exact identification of each bit of intelligence should then be printed neatly on the back in black marker.

We were to start this new program by preparing ten categories of bits of intelligence, each containing ten cards. Each category should be introduced joyfully to the child with an announcement such as, "Let's look at these salt water fish!" and then shown to the child at the same speed as the word cards—as fast as possible. Each category should be shown three times a day. Starting on the tenth day, the oldest card should be removed from each category, and a new one put in. Therefore, each card would be seen a total of 30 times before it was retired. When we ran out of bits for one particular category, we would retire the whole category and start a new category, adding and retiring after the tenth day. Bits must be shown at a happy time, not right after a fight. To solve a child's intelligence problem, he must be shown between 8,000 and 10,000 bits.

Later, Glenn Doman came back on the stage to tell us that actually we would only have to dream up and prepare nine categories of bits of intelligence because there was one particular ready-made category of 100 cards that could be purchased at the bookstore. The category was called instant math, and the cards were referred to as dot cards.

Each 11 x 11 inch card had on it from one to 100 randomly arranged ¾ -inch red dots. We were to show the first ten cards three times a day for ten days, and thenceforth remove two old cards a day and put in two new ones until all 100 had been seen 15 times (three times a day for five days), and then retire the last ten two at a time, taking five days. The total days required to thus present the 100 dot cards would be 60 days.

Before Doman started to describe the instant math program, he gave a sample dot card to a parent in the front row, with the instructions to quickly determine the number of dots in it, and then to pass it on to the next parent. When the card came to us, we became frustrated with counting and recounting the blur of red dots, and finally just guessed at the number. Doman later asked for everyone's answer. No one got it right. There were 78 dots, and, according to Doman, tiny children have the ability to recognize instantly the actual number of dots. They need only be told the name for each random configuration of dots, which was what we would be doing when presenting the dot cards as a category of bits.

In fact, tiny children can do addition, subtraction, multiplication, and division instantly, without doing it out the long way they are taught in school. We would teach our children to use this skill they already have by using the dot cards.

, On the back of each card are four equations. Twenty cards had four addition equations of increasing complexity, the particular dot card being the answer for each equation. For example, the card with seven red dots on the front had 3+4, 1+0+6, 1+2+1+3, and 2+1+2+1+1 on the back. Twenty different cards had four subtraction equations, also with an increasing number of steps, 20 had four division equations with an increasing number of steps, and 20 of the 100 dot cards had four mixed four-step equations, such as 20+4-8+2x5, 30+3x10-87+27, 42x2+6-10+2, 50+5x6+60-80, all equalling 40.

After the first 60 days of presenting the names for the random configurations of dots, we would then read from the back one of the addition equations and its answer while holding the dot side for Jamie to see. One equation constituted one math session. We would use ten different dot cards a day with addition problems and mark off which problem we presented. Once an equation was used, it was never repeated again that day or any day. The next day we would use ten more of the total of 80 addition problems in ten separate math sessions, and mark them off. Thus it would take eight days to be done with addition. Likewise, it would take eight days to go through the 80 subtraction problems, eight days for multiplication, eight days for division, and eight days for the mixed equations. In 40 days a child would have heard all 400 equations, completing the 100-day instant math program. The parents in the room were so astounded at this whole concept that they were unusually hushed and motionless.

Doman's final remarks concerned both reading and math. Our visual screen, explained our teacher, is very large. We should not have to read tiny word by tiny word, nor should we have to compute tiny dot by tiny dot. The human brain should be capable of taking in the whole two pages of an opened book or the whole card full of dots in the same way as it took in a whole scene out a window. In an instant we perceive the blue sky, the distant mountains, and the flowers in the field. We do not slowly "read" the scene, like dots that comprise a photograph, starting at the upper left and proceeding as if across a page. Blue, blue, blue. . . blue. Black, black (the mountains have started), blue, blue, black, black. . . . Black, black, blue, white, white (that's a cloud), blue, blue. . . . That is simply not the way the mind works. It sees all in a glance. So we should all be speed readers, and do math as instantly as a cheap plastic calculator. It is perhaps too late to retrain us as adults, but these were the goals we would pursue with our children. No one but Glenn Doman could have presented such unbelievable material so convincingly.

We had come to Philadelphia primarily with the hopes of getting Jamie to use his right hand. He was getting that and so much more. We thanked our lucky stars for leading us to Philadelphia, and marvelled that the rest of the world could be so critical. Why hadn't Doman won a Nobel Prize? We heard him say that his critics, when faced with one of his success stories, replied only that the dramatic changes in the child in question were due to factors such as natural maturation or increased parental attention, and not to the successful application of his theories. Such criticism prompted Doman to adopt a sarcastic motto for his Institutes: "Here is where what would have happened anyway happens!"

During the next two days we were informed what Jamie's new daily program should be. We were overwhelmed. It was so much more than the first program. That first program seemed overwhelming too in the beginning, but we had conquered it, I kept telling myself. This time not only was Jamie's daily work increased, but so was our nightly preparation, owing to the bits of intelligence program.

The only good news was a reduction in the number of maskings and cross patternings a day. Masking was reduced from 60 to 47 a day. Because of the heavier physical program, there wasn't as much time for masking. And we were to do four cross patterns instead of eight. That meant that Pattianne could go away to school in the fall without my having to find a replacement for her, that the many people who came twice a week would only have to come once.

Jamie was to continue crawling and creeping, but there was a new twist. In addition to long distance crawling and creeping, which was now referred to as marathon crawling and creeping, he was to do sprint crawling and creeping every day. He would work up to 15 ten-yard crawl sprints a day, with the goal of doing as many as possible of the 15 in less than 13 seconds each. And he would work up to 15 20-yard creep sprints a day, with the goal of doing as many as possible of those in less than 13 seconds each. His marathon crawling distance was the same as before, half a mile a day, but this time to be done in two 440-yard sessions, taking less than one hour total. Crawling could now be done on a rug, rather than on a smooth, hard surface, and he would be allowed to wear sneakers. His marathon creeping distance was halved to one mile per day, with the ultimate goal of doing 880 yards nonstop twice, and doing the whole mile in less than one hour. The purpose of all this creeping and crawling was to make Jamie a better walker, to improve visual convergence, to organize and grow his midbrain, and to actively stimulate his respiratory and vestibular systems.

Two more techniques would also actively stimulate Jamie's respiratory and vestibular systems. Brachiating and running. Instead of 30 single trips across the ladder a day, now Jamie was to do 30 round trips a day, which required learning to turn around in midair at the end of the ladder. In addition, he was to do two consecutive round trips a day nonstop by the time of the next visit. The purpose of brachiating, besides improving hand function in Jamie's particular case, was to improve and expand the structure of his chest and lungs to allow for deeper and more efficient respiration.

The new running program for Jamie was a third method of active vestibular stimulation, and of active respiratory patterning. Endurance running and sprint running both produced deep rhythmic breathing. Such breathing supplied the brain with more oxygen, which was necessary to organize the cortex and to improve all neurological functions.

Jamie's ultimate goal was to run three miles a day nonstop in less than 46 minutes! To a non-jogging family, both the distance and the time were a shock. He would work up to the three miles following a precise schedule of increases that would take ten weeks. Alden had a bum hip and could not possibly run. I knew who would be following the precise schedule of buildup along with Jamie. Me. I was a swimmer, skier, golfer, and sailor, but not a runner. Jogging was the current craze, but it had never appealed to me. Now I would be forced into it.

In addition to the long distance running, Jamie was assigned 20 30-yard running sprints a day, with the goal of doing as many as possible in less than five seconds each. As with creeping and crawling, we were to record all times and distances daily. In addition to that record, we were to compute the average time for the creep sprints, the crawl sprints, and the running sprints per day. With 15 creep sprints, 15 crawl sprints, and 20 running sprints a day, that was a lot of math. If only someone had shown me the dot cards when I was young so I could do instant math! And we were to send a picture to our advocate of Jamie running by September 3.

Though we were stunned by the doubled brachiation and the addition of running and sprints, we were relieved to learn that we would not be required to implement any passive vestibular stimulation. No twirling upside down for Jamie. That had been my greatest fear for two days. They had decided that active vestibular activities, particularly brachiating and running, were sufficient at this time.

Next we learned how to do passive respiratory patterning on Jamie. He lay on a patterning table with the vest on, its long straps leading to dowels on either side of him. Alden and I sat on opposite sides of the table and practiced pulling the dowels that in turn tightened the vest on Jamie's chest, and releasing them, all to the steady beat of the metronome. Twenty breaths per minute, one beat for inspiring and two beats for expiring. Three beats per breath. We were to set the metronome for 60 beats per minute and to do respiratory patterning three times a day for 20 minutes each time. I could see that it would be a relaxing 20 minutes, and I welcomed it. After we were pronounced perfect at it, we expected the instructor to give us the vest and send us to our next appointment. Instead she handed us complex instruction sheets on how to sew up the vest at home, with the added hint that we could purchase the metronome, the canvas, the padding, the D ring, the heavy thread, the rubber washers, and the two wooden dowels at the Institutes' bookstore! I just happened to have a sewing machine and I just happened to be fairly skilled at using it. But what were less fortunate mothers to do?

Our last appointment came early Friday afternoon, right after a short meeting with the pediatrician who prescribed the same vitamin regimen as before. It was with a person from the Institute for the Achievement of Intellectual Excellence. She described Jamie's reading, writing, spelling, math, and bits of intelligence program. I was to continue showing Jamie ten categories of ten words three times each day, with ten old cards retired a day and ten new cards added a day. And I was to continue making brief homemade books to read to him, but instead of a new one every week, I was to prepare a new one every day. In addition, I was to teach him to write and spell three words a week. These sessions should not last more than 30 seconds and should be used as a treat after he had done something well. Finally, she reviewed the bits of intelligence and math programs that we had learned about in the lectures. Ten categories of ten cards, shown three times a day, one card from each category or one whole category retired a day, and ten new cards added a day. The dot cards would be one category. The other nine categories should be as sophisticated as possible to insure that Jamie was receiving new information.

We went to the bookstore to purchase the math kit, several bottles of vitamins, the metronome, and the materials for the respiratory vest. I also bought several copies of a paperback book to circulate among my volunteers. It was written by a parent of a brain-injured child and explained the philosophy and program of the Institutes in concise form. I also bought, for the benefit of my helpers, several postcards showing the beautiful grounds and buildings of the Institutes. These I would mount on a poster and display in the patterning room. And I bought two packets of picture cards they happened to have—house plants and musical composers. All I had to do was mount them. Our total bill for this stop was over $100.

Since it was only 2:00 p.m. after we paid our monthly bill in the business office and picked up our new box of masks, we decided to go back to Guilene's, pack up our things, and leave right away. We knew we couldn't afford to waste any time. We were in our own beds by midnight and spent Saturday preparing for Jamie's new program.

20
I Will Survive

They expect tots to absorb Bach or Van Gogh before solid food.
Langway, 1983, p. 62

Before going to Philadelphia a second time, since we knew the basics, the thought had crept into our minds that we could just continue on our own without having to pay $250 a month. Jamie could creep and crawl and brachiate and be cross patterned until he was well.

But now we knew the value of revisits. We would never have thought of respiratory patterning. We would never have thought of sprints. We would never have thought of bits. Or round trip brachiating. Or running. We definitely needed Glenn Doman's guidance, inventiveness, and enthusiasm.

Saturday morning we waited for the department stores and bookstores to open so that I could comb them for decent jogging shoes for Jamie and myself, large quantities of poster board, rubber cement, markers, and picture books suitable for bits. While we waited, Alden and I rearranged the living room furniture. Jamie needed a straight 10-yard and 20-yard course for indoor crawling and creeping sprints. That meant we had to move the couch away from the wall that led into the hall. The combined distance of the length of the hallway and the living room was exactly ten yards. That was perfect for sprint crawling and a round trip was perfect for sprint creeping. We had only to figure out how to put more pieces in less space. An hour of trial and error resulted in an arrangement along three walls that was reasonably attractive. I didn't particularly like the bare fourth wall in the living room, but I could live with it if it would help make my son well.

Later, at the mall, I went to the grocery and department stores and bought everything we needed, including several large picture books of reptiles, breeds of dogs, breeds of cats, antique autos, types of guns, famous paintings, and seashells. I also bought a 12-foot piece of four-inch foam, and fabric with which to cover it. This was to put under the ladder. Now that Jamie was on the verge of independent brachiating, I wanted to protect him during his inevitable falls. I remembered that only a few nights before our trip to Philadelphia Jamie had been determined to show Judi and her family how he could go all the way across the ladder alone. Judi brought supper over, as she frequently did, and we were all sitting at the picnic table by the pool, when Jamie suddenly got up and said, "Watch this!" He had gone only half way when, to my horror, he suddenly fell to the ground hard on his back. I vowed at that moment to get a pad and to always stand by him when he was using the ladder, lest we find ourselves returning to the Institutes with a more seriously brain injured child than we already had.

The total cost of my afternoon at the mall was $200. That evening, as Alden began cutting the expensive books and I began cutting the canvas for the respiratory vest, we discussed our finances. Our reduced savings account would not cover the three more monthly payments we were responsible for before we returned to Philadelphia in November. We had already paid the Institutes $1,450—$450 for the initial evaluation and $250 a month for four months. Related expenses had amounted so far to almost $1,000—lumber, masonite, newspaper ads, hotel and meals and tolls, subscriptions, the masks I had ordered on my own before April, timers and counters and a stopwatch, a wall clock, poster board, markers, vitamins, math kit, metronome, respiratory vest, books (some to be read and some to be mutilated), and two pairs of running shoes.

Some parents told us that they had not paid the Institutes a cent. They were waiting for results first. Our consciences would not allow us to do that. We had agreed to pay and we would. But we had to find a way to meet our obligation to the Institutes. We made a grave decision that Saturday night. We would close out the children's savings accounts. The accounts were very small and we never added to them. I had opened them as each child had been born, and had deposited money they had received from relatives and friends. The combined total was almost $250—just enough to meet September's payment. We suppressed our guilt with a promise to pay them back, and returned to our cutting.

Sunday, August 17, we resumed the program. It was Day 102. Alden and I worked together with Jamie that Sunday, but Alden decided that from then on he and Dick would run the program on weekends, leaving me free to get some of the night work done in the daytime. Except for bits and respiratory patterning, neither of which we were yet prepared to do, Jamie met all his goals (distance, not speed) scheduled for that day. He actually exceeded the running goal. He was to do only 220 yards at a time, 20 times. But I couldn't stop him! He loved it! He would run the 220 yards Alden had measured on the road in front of our house six or seven times before I could make him stop for a while. I was huffing and stopped long before he did. My little spiral notebook looked like this at the end of the day.

New Program   Day 102
Sunday, August 17

Bits	—Not ready	
RP	—vest not made	(respiratory patterning)
XP	—1 2 3 4	(cross patterning)
br	—20 rt (with help)	(brachiating—round trips)
m	—47	(masking)
cr	—880/25; 880/40	(creeping—yd/min.)
s cr	—20/15; 20/16; 20/15; 20/16	(sprint creeping—yd/sec.)
cw	—440/40; 440/55	(crawling—yd/min.)
s cw	—10/15; 10/16; 10/13; 10/13; 10/13	(sprint crawling—yd/sec.)
s r	—20/6; 20/6; 20/7; 20/6; 20/6	(sprint running—yd/sec.)
r	—1320/14; 880/10; 1540/17; 1540/20	(running—yd/min.)

On the blue sheets that I would be returning to the Institutes with our lengthy interim report, I entered the totals for marathon crawling, creeping, and running—880 yards in 95 minutes, 1,760 yards in 55 minutes, and three miles in 61 minutes, respectively. For each of the three kinds of sprints, I had to enter the best time and the average time.

I was elated that Jamie seemed to do so well. All he had to do was to improve his time and work up to the full number of brachiates and sprints. All I had to do was finish the vest and come up with enough bits for ten new ones a day and keep the log. I thought I could do it. That was a definite improvement in my attitude as compared to my negativism when I had been faced with the first program the Institutes had assigned us back in April. Jamie was going to win—I would make it happen.

There was so much busy work this time that there was no time for anything else. The beans in our garden grew big and tough and we never picked them. The tomatoes dropped from the vines. The program had already proven to be a reliable method of birth control the last time, but it was even more reliable this time. We worked hard all day and then labored all evening on word cards and bits of intelligence cards. When we went to bed it was vital to get a good night's sleep before the 5:30 alarm forced us back into the therapy room again. Occasionally Alden and I passed unexpectedly in the hallway, paused for a brief passionate kiss, and then went on with the program.

By Wednesday night, after four nights of staying up until after midnight, I had the respiratory vest ready to use, though I still hadn't finished quilting it. On Tuesday afternoon, Cora Jo had turned all nine of the 30-inch straps right side out for me, a time-consuming and tedious job, so that I just had to sew them to the body of the vest that night in order to make it operational. From then on, Alden and I did one respiratory patterning at

6:00 a.m. and one some time after work, and I did one with a volunteer at midday. I taught six people how to do it—Anita, Jane, Pierra, Darlene, Dixie, and Jeanne. I explained to them all about Karen Ann Quinlan, and hung the "Vital Statements and Rules of the Respiratory Program," a green sheet given us by the Institutes, on the wall. It said, in short, that one of the people patterning must be a parent of the child, that if the child was sick, respiratory patterning must be discontinued until he was well, that if a parent was apprehensive about any aspect of this patterning it must be halted and the Institutes notified, that it was the parents' responsibility to teach and to caution volunteers about respiratory patterning, that the child should have no food or small objects in front of his face while being patterned, and that no mechanical or electrical devices should be used in place of people to do the patterning. There was another green sheet that I was instructed to post as well. It described the proper sitting position, the proper way to pull on the straps, and emphasized that there must be no talking and no distractions while executing respiratory patterning. I hung both papers right under the colorful postcards of the Institutes.

I needed more help than ever from my volunteers. Not only for cross patterning and respiratory patterning, but I depended on them heavily as well to cut and paste bits. I managed to have the first 100 cards ready by the second Monday, but after ten days I needed ten new ones every day. Not to mention ten reading words a day and one new homemade book a day. Just measuring and cutting up the poster board for all this was a job in itself.

I decided on my own to make bits 9 x 11 inches instead of the prescribed 11 x 11 inches because that way I could get six cards per 28 x 22 inch piece of poster board instead of only four. Economy was an important factor in our lives.

Jane picked up package after package of poster board for me as she had before. She and Anita did most of the measuring and cutting for my three different uses. Others cut, labeled, and glued pictures from the books I bought and from posters and booklets I had ordered and was receiving daily. The book of shells that I had bought would last as a category for many months. I hoped that Jamie would not become too bored with conches, cowries, and clams. Also I had a large world map that Anita cut into individual counties for me to mount. And I had a poster of the corresponding national flags. The shells, the countries, the flags, the cards of houseplants that I had bought at the Institutes, along with the dot cards, made up five of the ten required categories. These five categories would each last a long time before being exhausted. So I really only had to worry about five other categories for a while.

Over the weeks, my volunteers were extremely helpful in thinking up new categories for me, and finding the appropriate magazine pictures—types of architecture, musical instruments, political leaders, entertainers, sports activities. Susan's mother, a retired teacher, donated a set of pictures of wild flowers already mounted; Judi, a Lamaze instructor, made a set of cards showing the internal sequence of reproduction from fertilization to birth; her husband made a set of the different constellations; Jane drew road signs and animal footprints and parts of a horse. We could never have come up with all the ideas, or the time, on our own.

With my eyes watchful for bits in the magazines my friends contributed by the boxful, I once spotted a picture that I knew deserved to be displayed on our refrigerator. It showed a harried father holding a screaming and flailing infant in one arm, and mixing up a meal with the other hand, and a five-year-old daughter tugging at his belt. It was perfect and Alden managed to smile at it when I taped it in place.

Summer ended abruptly, as usual. The nights were cold beginning in August, and by early September the pool temperature had dropped from 80 degrees to 60 degrees. I was glad. If I didn't have time to swim, then I didn't want anyone else to be able to either. Alden was similarly cynical. He longed for the first snow to end the golfing season so that his buddies couldn't play any more. It was now barely light when we rose at 5:30. I hated that hour, but since this program took so much longer, if we didn't get the early start, it would be impossible to finish.

Just before school was due to reopen, Alden and I, armed with a support letter of medical exemption from the Institutes, had a meeting with the principal, the school nurse, and the school guidance counselor to request permission to keep Jamie out of first grade. It was easier than we anticipated. The law in Maine did not require a child to go to school until he was seven. Jamie was 6 / and it was our prerogative to keep him home. The nurse and the counselor inquired with enthusiasm about the program, and in general were very supportive. The new principal, on the other hand, had a doubting look and a condescending attitude. Her only comment after listening to our description of the rigid demands and long hours of the program was, "And may I ask where is Jamieson at this moment?" As if he were loafing and we were liars. I explained that Anita, my most experienced volunteer, was timing his creeping and crawling while we had to be away for a short while.

Having gotten over the hurdle of keeping Jamie out of school, we then made a bolder request. Since it had already been written into his special education plan last spring that he still needed an aide in the classroom, and since this aide, Lynne (one of our volunteers since May), had already been rehired for the current school year, couldn't she be permitted to come to our house to perform her duties? The nurse and counselor thought it was an excellent idea. The principal coldly stated that the decision would have to be made by the superintendent, and that she would let me know.

The first day of school arrived. Jennifer had been excited about kindergarten for weeks. She was more attached to me than Jamie had been, but I think that she would have been willing to go anywhere just to get out of the house and away from the program. Earlier in the summer, she had consented to going home with Grampa one night, and home with Susan another night—both trips causing Jamie extreme jealousy and me extreme surprise because never before had she been brave enough to leave me, though she had often been offered the opportunity. She was showing no signs of hesitation this morning either.

We waited out front for the bus. Jennifer had on a new dress and carried Jamie's old lunch box for her morning snack. Jamie, not aware of his own hostility about yet another trip he was being denied, said in an innocent voice, "Wouldn't it be too bad if the big yellow bus forgot to stop?" I cried for the second year in a row when the bus did stop. But my tears this year were not only for the child that was so easily leaving me, but also for the one staying behind, shivering beside me in his bare feet and knee pads. As I put my camera away, I silently vowed, "Next year, baby, you'll go to school too, I promise!"

The days went by, and Jamie's running steadily improved. The first few days on the new program he had tried to do too much too fast and I had mistakenly let him. His leg muscles had soon been sore, and he had been barely able to run. But by the time Jennifer started school, he had sufficiently recovered so that instead of running one mile three separate times during the day, we were running three miles nonstop. We made our best time when we ran by a house that had a dog. Jamie was deathly afraid of barking dogs and I couldn't convince him that their barks were friendly. He ran so fast that I couldn't catch him when he was passing a house where a dog was protecting his territory. He ran equally fast past homes where a dog had once barked at us, but was not even in sight now. I was tempted, in the interest of speed, to call my neighbors and ask them to make sure that their pets were outside at 5:00 each afternoon, but decided that Jamie's nerves couldn't take it.

Several of our friends who were runners had told us how addicting it was. It was a national craze. There were joggers everywhere at all times in various getups. I was in shape and I knew that I could easily do the three required miles at a much faster pace than I did with Jamie, or do more than three miles if I were so inclined. But there was one problem—I was not so inclined. In fact, it was worse than that. I could never say it out loud or in front of Jamie, but late at night, in the dark, I admitted to Alden my innermost feelings. I hated to run!

How could so many people choose to do it day after day after day? I now knew how Jamie felt when he was counting laps while creeping and crawling and was constantly asking, "What number am I on?" He needed to know how close to the end he was. I had the same need when running.

I found I had the road all divided up. If I could just endure it to that telephone pole, I would have only one more mile to go, and at the corner I had it made—a quarter of a mile until my front doorstep. I was even mentally keeping track of how many more total miles I had left to run before our week "vacation" in Philadelphia.

To my great relief, Aunt Susie ran with Jamie on Saturdays and Uncle Dick ran with him on Sundays. Dick and Susan were more openly vocal about their dislike of running than I could afford to be. I couldn't take the chance of negatively influencing Jamie's attitude toward a required exercise. But Dick and Susan could moan and groan in pain, and Jamie thought it was great fun to be the cause of such torture. It was undoubtedly a more grueling exertion for Dick and Susan because they each ran only once a week and not at all in between. Susan once confided to me that when she ran with Jamie she fantasized that over each hill would be me, in the big yellow convertible, waiting to pick her up.

I was surprised one day to find four sets of theatre tickets in my mailbox. We had been enthusiastic season's subscribers to Theatre by the Sea in Portsmouth for several years, and had decided the previous spring to renew our subscription as usual for the following winter season despite the financial and physical demands of the program. But why had they sent us four reserved seats for each production instead of two? I looked through my checkbook record, and found that I had indeed paid for the two subscriptions twice. With so much on my mind, and with so many new expenses, I had probably received a circular from the theater encouraging membership after I had already renewed, and just renewed again without even remembering the prior renewal. I was embarrassed at this slip-up. What was happening to my usual obnoxious efficiency?

We decided that since we had already paid for them, the tickets would be useful as gifts to our most dedicated volunteers. And it would be fun to have company every time we went to a performance.

A few mornings later, when Alden and I were doing the first respiratory patterning of the day on Jamie, Alden suddenly noted, "Hey, it's awfully quiet in here." To my blank stare he said, "You forgot to turn on the metronome!" I just heard the click so clearly and evenly in my head all the time that I hadn't even noticed that the real thing was missing.

That night I was tired and silly when we were doing the last respiratory patterning of the day. Benji was standing beside me and needed to be entertained as he leaned on my thigh. So I began to blow bubbles for him. With my own saliva. After all, my hands were busy. Alden thought it was repulsive, from the look on his face, but refrained from comment until I had missed a beat of the metronome four times. Then he blurted out, "I don't mind your spitting all over the place, but would you please pay attention to the metronome!"

The very next day, when I was upstairs fixing a cup of coffee for one of the volunteers while Jamie crawled in the kitchen between patterns, I put the hot coffee pot in the refrigerator after pouring the hot water into the cup, and then put the plastic jug of milk on the hot burner! I was sitting on the floor admonishing Jamie to speed it up when I smelled the burning polyethylene and heard the glugging of leaking milk.

With all these events, I began to doubt myself. Was I cracking up? I jokingly told everyone I was near a breakdown. I was playfully exaggerating, but nevertheless, on one of my rare trips off the property I bought a large button that declared, I WILL SURVIVE. Sometimes I wore it, and sometimes Jamie wore it.

Dick helped me to preserve my sanity a little when he showed up the first weekend in October with a bicycle for me. He had picked it up at a yard sale for his mother, but she never used it. He had seen it in the cellar and had a brainstorm. I could pedal instead of pound beside Jamie! It was one of Dick's better ideas.

I explained to Jamie that he was too fast for an old girl like me and that my knees kept giving out (which in fact they did, though not severely enough or often enough to justify quitting running). He accepted this new arrangement. He probably figured that anything that came from Uncle Dick was okay. I gleefully mounted by new blue lifesaver, secure in the knowledge that I would never run again. My survival was now guaranteed a little longer.

21
Of Frogs and Farts

It is crucial to know if the child's growth is generalizable to broader areas of behavior not measured by the Profile.

Zigler and Sparrow, 1978, p. 139

The philodendron plants in the long planter between the kitchen and the living room began to die. They could survive a certain amount of neglect—sporadic feeding and lack of sunlight, but they apparently could not survive outright abuse. I had for weeks kept hundreds of word cards and picture cards and dot cards balanced atop the planter in which the philodendron struggled to grow. There the cards were safe, and yet handy. On the kitchen counter they would get wet; on any of the tables they would have to be continually moved; in boxes or closets they would be inaccessible. Starting at one end of the planter and working toward the center, first there was a pile of 100 bits to be shown that day; next was the spot to pile those same bits as each category was shown, next was the pile of 100 word cards for the day, and beside that was the spot to pile those after they were shown, and finally came the homemade story for the day. Starting at the other end of the planter and working toward the center, there was the pile of newly-made bits waiting to be activated; then a similar pile of word cards; then came the dots; and finally a pile of blank cards of assorted sizes. In between all these peeked desperate sprigs of heart-shaped green leaves. Their final doom was sealed when I gave up watering them to preserve the undersides of my precious cards from being splattered with wet soil.

I believed in the single word cards. They had greatly contributed to teaching Jamie to read in the first place, and now continued to be useful to teach him more words. But I was skeptical about the daily homemade books. Now that Jamie was an eager reader, they were too simple. He craved more complex reading material. Dixie still came to help us one day a week, after her teaching duties. As she was now a first grade teacher, she loaned me, with the school's approval, all the first grade texts and workbooks. She monitored his reading and other academic progress. She listened to Jamie read and judged him to be far ahead of her first grade class.

My belief in the bits of intelligence cards was at first somewhat less than firm. I showed them at high speed and was never supposed to test Jamie. All that work and expense and I had no idea what he was retaining. He did immensely enjoy each session though, and so did Jennifer. She requested to be notified whenever I was going to show a pack so that she too could be present. She came on the run, paused to look and listen for ten seconds, and then resumed her previous activity. Occasionally I did get some unexpected feedback that bolstered my commitment. When the fall weeds were in full bloom in our back yard, Jennifer announced confidently that they were New England Asters. I, who had only seen the backs of cards as I flipped through them, ran for my pack of wild flowers to corroborate her declaration. She was right. And Jamie told me one day that the stop sign that he ran to every day was shaped like an octagon, not only correctly recalling one of the shapes in the geometric designs that I had drawn, but generalizing it to a more concrete object in his environment. My faith in the bits grew.

I was definitely skeptical about the dot cards. I hesitated to tell just anyone about the instant math program. It was too wacky if one was not into all this as deeply as we were. Yet people saw the cards and wanted to know about them. I could tell by the expressions on their faces that my quick explanation and mock enthusiasm were insufficient to convince laymen. Yet I really did want to convince them and myself because damaged credibility for one aspect of the program meant damaged credibility for other aspects of the program.

We had been warned at the Institutes that infants learn instant math easily, but that it might be too late for a six-year-old, because he had already been exposed to conventional numbers and operations. We should try it anyway for a while in case Jamie's brain was still receptive to it.

Jamie stared obediently at the blur of red dots, but showed no sign of being able to discern 78 of them from 82 of them. His interest perked up a little when I began reciting equations to him after the first 60 days. When I held up the card with 20 dots on it and said that $2 \times 10 = 20$, he replied that $5 + 5 + 5 + 5$ was also 20. When I showed him nine dots and said that $90 \div 2 + 1 + 5 + 1 = 9$, he replied that $3 + 3 + 3$ was also 9, and in fact that $5 + 4$ was 9 too—as if to say there was an easier way to get 9!

Independent brachiation was the most difficult goal to achieve. On Friday of the first week of the new program, Jamie had done three round trips alone. We had gone to the tires playground for a few minutes as a reward. The following Sunday he had done eleven round trips alone and earned a trip to the pier to gaze at Uncle Dick's sailboat. After that, his hands had been so sore and red that I had been barely able to persuade him to do one a day alone for the next three weeks. Alden and I supported most of his weight as he did his 30 round trips. He cried almost every day from the pain of the open sores on his palms and fingers, caused by friction with the rungs when I would swing his body, as instructed, to get the momentum to glide to the next rung. His left shoulder, which did most of the work whenever I lessened my support for a few seconds, ached too.

Again I was tempted to give it up and quit torturing an innocent child. But just in time I saw that the sores were healing and turning to hard callouses. So I offered him the ultimate incentive. When he did 15 round trips alone he could have the rest of the day off. A few days later, as he was finishing his last brachiate of the day at 8:00 p.m.—only his tenth without help—he said, "Only five more would have been 15. Tomorrow I will do 15 alone—early!" He knew that the reward would be greater the sooner he fulfilled the requirement.

Sure enough, by 7:00 a.m. the following morning he had already done five alone—along with 900 yards of creeping, one respiratory patterning, five brachiates with support, several maskings, and several intelligence sessions.

Though the pain was diminished, each round trip on the ladder still required nearly superhuman effort. He did it slowly and jerkily. His right hand reached forward awkwardly, and then, after a pause, his left hand shot forward at lightning speed, before the lesser grip of the right hand could fail to support his weight. It was particularly difficult for him to muster up enough momentum to do the turn-around in midair at the end of the ladder. It made me tense to watch the whole procedure. He could not do more than two, or at most three, consecutive round trips. Then he needed to rest. By rest, I mean he did other program things.

At 3:00 p.m., Jamie did his 15th independent brachiation, and went off joyously to do as he pleased for the remainder of the afternoon and evening. It was Day 130. It happened to be Sunday, so I didn't have to cancel the arrival of any patterners. Daddy and Uncle Dick took him fishing and out for a hot dog, and I relaxed with Susan like old times.

Jamie desperately wanted to do all 30 brachiates without help, not only because I had promised him that he could quit at one o'clock on the Sunday following that achievement (Sunday so that we could celebrate all together as a family, and with Susan and Dick too), but also because he felt satisfaction in meeting the prescribed goals. He had the strength and the will, but his hands were sore again. For several days he could not do more than ten to 15 alone. But for the first time he was confident in his ability, and every day he showed the volunteers who came to our house that he could brachiate. I had been telling them that he could, but not one had ever witnessed it. Now they finally believed me, and were amazed and proud along with me.

On Day 139 Jamie did all 30 round trip brachiates independently! He wasn't able to do it again for several days. But I knew that soon he would do them all alone every day, and also be strong enough to do two consecutive round trips without stopping, as directed by the Institutes. The following Sunday, Jamie reaped his reward. It was a clear and warm fall day, and we went sailing on Dick's boat. I put away the timer and the clickers and packed supper in the cooler. It felt strange to do something so normal.

As I allowed myself the luxury of closing my eyes while lying on the deck, a startling thought occurred to me. All this work for the past seven months had been merely preparation for the procedure that might ultimately cure Jamie. Carrying him under the ladder would never cure his bent hand, but supporting his own weight with that hand might. We were just barely to the point where he could brachiate alone, and it was that independent brachiation, repeated day in and day out, for an as yet undetermined length of time that was in our estimation vital to Jamie's getting well. We hadn't really made any significant progress yet. The next six months should reveal the possibilities to us. I wanted to share these thoughts with Alden, but he was manning the jib sheets, and since we were tacking our way out of the harbor, he was busy. "Ready, about!" shouted Captain Hobson, and I put my head down to avoid being hit by the boom, and saved my thoughts till later.

Jamie felt so good about his proven ability as a runner, a reader, and a brachiator that his attitude toward even the debasing and tedious crawling and creeping began to improve. I guess he figured he should do that well too. He moved faster than I had ever thought was possible. He consistently did each of his 240-yard marathon crawls in 20 to 25 minutes, easily reaching the goal of a half a mile in less than one hour. After he came upstairs from working with Daddy each morning, he ate breakfast and then did 440 yards of crawling. If he finished before 8:00, I allowed him to go outside with Jennifer to wait for the bus. Some other children also got on at our house, so it was a chance for him to socialize too. All I had to say as he crawled down the hall or around the kitchen table was, "Jamie, the bus comes in five minutes," and he moved like lightning. Likewise, his two 900-yard marathon creeps were each done in 20 to 25 minutes, also beating the one hour maximum for the whole mile. Formerly he had lazily done only half as much in the same time.

By mid-September, Jamie's daily schedule was as follows:

5:30-6:00	dressed, 3 masks, juice, fruit, vitamins, bits, words
6:00-6:20	respiratory patterning with Daddy
6:20-7:15	5 round trip brachiates, 900 yards creeping, masking (with Daddy)
7:15-7:30	breakfast, bits, words
7:30-7:55	440 yards crawling
7:55-8:10	outside break
8:10-8:30	5 round trip brachiates, bits, words, writing, masking
8:30-9:00	15 creeping sprints
9:00-10:00	2 cross patterns, run 3 miles

10:00-12:00	10 round trip brachiates, 900 yards creeping, 15 crawl sprints, masking, snack, bits, words, book
12:00-1:00	2 cross patterns, 1 respiratory pattern, 5 brachiates, masking
1:00-1:30	lunch, break, masking, bits, words
1:30-3:00	440 yards crawling, 5 brachiates, 15 running sprints, masking
3:00-4:40	time off, if it was a good day, or finish up if it was slow
4:40-5:00	last respiratory patterning with Daddy

Most days went smoothly and I seldom had to use force with Jamie. He was a conquered soul and I was the robot who drove him. We never worked until 8:00 or 9:00 at night any more as in the very beginning, except sometimes on the weekends when Daddy and Dick were on duty and goofed off too much all day. I was the only one compulsive enough to stick to a schedule. I had to be rigid because I needed the evenings to complete the lengthy midterm and end of term reports. I was very descriptive and positive when answering all the questions about Jamie's progress because I was pleased.

But I cheated on two sections of the report. I was supposed to compute the average sprint times from the 15 separate times he sprint crawled, from the 15 separate times he sprint crept, and from the 15 separate times he sprint ran. That was too much computation for me, even with a calculator. I had all the individual times recorded in my notebook, but I just guessed at the averages. I doubted that anyone at the Institutes would check my math. What did it matter what his average was? I had enough to do without spending all night adding and dividing.

The other shortcut I took was on the diet sheet. Ever since we had first applied to the Institutes I had been filling out their diet sheet whenever they wanted it with disgusting faithfulness. It was two pages long and required that I not only keep track of every morsel that passed Jamie's lips for breakfast, lunch, dinner, and snacks for seven days, but how much each morsel weighed, how many grams of protein it contained, and the time it was consumed! I'd had several copies made of the last one that I had diligently computed, and now I just pulled one from my file and placed it without the slightest twinge of guilt in the appropriate spot in the report.

A few days later we got a short note back from our advocate. It was congratulatory and my shortcuts had not been detected. But we were appalled at the request for even more detail and computation.

Dear Mr. and Mrs. Bratt,
Thank you for your interim report. From all indications you are doing a terrific job. The changes in Jamieson sound superb.

The only request I have is that you be more specific about the quantity of Jamieson's reading program. Please be prepared to tell us exactly how many words, sentences and books he has seen this period.

My best to you all and special congratulations to Jamieson.

Keep up the good work.

In October Jennifer had a Halloween birthday party. I went out of my way to be sure that I gave her enough extra attention on her special day, as if I could make up for lost time with her all at once. She seemed moody lately, or "reserved," as her kindergarten teacher described her. She openly resented the praise we lavished on Jamie as he met more and more of his goals. Her birthday was luckily on a Saturday, so I was all hers. Jennifer and I went to the store for party supplies and three goldfish. She knew better than to ask for a more demanding or expensive pet. The largest and most shimmering of the three she named Jello.

Benjiman, on the other hand, didn't seem to ever mind the program. He wasn't even aware that there was such a thing as a time before the program. He would be shocked when he went to school and found out from his friends that other families didn't creep and crawl and brachiate and pattern all day. Of course Benjiman crept well now. He thought it was a lark to follow along behind Jamie and didn't even mind it when Jamie turned around and knocked him down while rushing by on his return trip down the hall.

I was tired from late nights and early mornings and exhausting days. I took all the vitamins that Jamie took. They helped to keep me going. I was also tired from an increased number of afternoons and evenings out. Such outings were supposed to relax me and make me better able to tackle the next day's responsibilities. But sometimes we stayed out too late, or when we came back I went straight to the scissors and glue to work on the bits that I felt guilty about not having done earlier that night.

I was tired of trying to make ends meet. We had met September's payment to the Institutes by closing the children's savings accounts. We met October's payment by selling my deceased mother's Hammond organ through an ad in the paper. Though I couldn't play it, it had been dear to me—but it had to go. To meet November's payment, we sold the bar and its two stools from the TV room, some silverware that had belonged to Alden's mother, and four of my mother's rings. We didn't speak about these sales to anyone, and we hardly spoke to each other about them. We had now spent over $3,000 on the program. Alden sarcastically admonished me to refrain from paying any bills twice, remembering our four season's tickets to Theatre by the Sea. Christmas was coming and we feared that it would be a meager one. Would the expenses ever cease? Would the long hours ever cease? Would the exhaustion ever cease?

One rainy day, I stared for a long time through the kitchen sliding glass door at a large bullfrog trying repeatedly and patiently to climb to freedom up the slippery side of the vinyl pool cover, which dipped down to the now only half-filled pool and was anchored by water bags up on the brick patio. The frog's struggle with life was akin to ours, I thought. He faced an unsurmountable obstacle, but he wouldn't give up. I also noted that the frog had perfect cross pattern motion.

Just two weeks before we were to return to Philadelphia for the third time, we received a little support for our cause when we were informed that it had been approved for the school aide to come to our house a short time each day. It was not for as many hours as I had hoped, but it would nevertheless be a great help. The best part was that it would be our friend Lynne coming to our house, and not another stranger we would have to acclimate to our routine. Lynne was easy to have around and had a strong rapport with Jamie. She was soft-spoken, yet firm and dedicated. She never yelled, yet never lost control of Jamie.

It was Day 165 of the program when Lynne started. We had managed for 164 days without her, but there were several reasons why I needed her. Jamie needed a break from the constant sound of my voice, and I needed some time during the day to do some bits and word cards, thus lessening my evening chores. Lynne's involvement also offered security against the next program. Though we were finishing early now, we fully expected the experts (or fanatics) in Philadelphia to double everything after Jamie's reevaluation. Then we would need Lynne more than ever.

But the very best reason for having Lynne relieve me for a while was Benjiman. He always miraculously slept through my 5:30 arousal of Jamie, and even when I awoke Jennifer a little after 7:00. He woke up conveniently at 8:30, and then I needed to change and feed him. I generally had Jamie doing timed sprints up and down the hall at that time. So as I removed Benjiman's sleeper every morning on the changing table in the bathroom, I yelled loudly, so Jamie could hear me at the other end of the hall, "Ready, set, go!" As Jamie pounded at top speed, and as I continued to wipe and powder, I estimated the elapsed seconds, "One...two...three...four... ." I knew when to stop counting because Jamie yelled "Done" and the thumping stopped. I mentally kept track of the times for six to eight sprints until I could write them down when I left the bathroom. The only trouble was that Benjiman probably thought that all this was perfectly normal, and would grow up to change his own child's pants yelling, "Ready, set, go!"

Now with Lynne quietly organizing and timing the sprints, I looked straight at Benjiman as I dressed him, and later as I fed him, I cooed softly to him. He seemed in a state of disbelief for a few days, but then clearly enjoyed the new attention.

The last day of our current program finally arrived. It was Friday,

October 31, Day 176 for us, Day 355 for the Iranian hostages. It was 6:10 a.m. and Jamie was lying on his back on the patterning table as Alden and I did the first respiratory patterning of the day. I had taken Jamie and Jennifer trick-or-treating the night before. Jamie had been as disoriented and spacey as ever in finding his way to the front doors and back to the car. Once back home, both had overdosed on the forbidden sweets.

Now, as Alden and I rhythmically pulled and released the straps that led to the respiratory vest on Jamie's chest, to the unerring beat of the metronome, Jamie was having a problem with lower intestinal tract gas. Too much chocolate, I told myself, trying to avoid eye contact with my husband. Otherwise I was afraid I would giggle, and sobriety on this matter was preferable in front of Jamie. Finally, Alden, arch-supporter of the Institutes' program to our friends and relatives, could take it no longer, and declared, with a straight face that didn't fool even Jamie, "This is Glenn Doman's fart machine, owned and operated by the fools who believe in the program. Let's squeeze a little harder and see if we can get another one out."

We spent so much time being dedicated and serious that it felt good to be a little human, too. Not only were we allowing ourselves to express a mild vulgarity, but we were also allowing ourselves to express the pent-up doubt that was inevitable with such a program, even in the face of so much progress.

22
Third Visit

It is not my intention to try to inflict my opinions on anyone else.
                                    Melton, 1972, p. 173

We were taking a day off before driving to Philadelphia. We drove the short distance to Susan's on Saturday, and from there we all went into Boston to the Museum of Fine Arts for the afternoon. We had made several delightful trips with Jamie and Jennifer to the Aquarium and the Children's Museum in Boston before the program. But I felt that it would be worthwhile to do something more worldly, especially since I had shown the kids so many bits of paintings and sculptures.

As we walked from room to room, we admired ancient pottery and jewelry, and stone sculptures. One could almost sense the great pyramids. Jennifer particularly liked the statue of "King Mycerinus and His Wife." In another room, we looked at paintings by French impressionists. Jamie ran right over to one and said, "That's 'The Carriage at the Races' by Degas!" I was bursting with pride and Alden and Susan were astounded. On another wall Jamie pointed to a painting he had never seen and said, "That one looks like how Monet painted." The little brass plate verified that Monet was indeed the artist. And then Jamie noticed a nearby painting and correctly identified it as "Rouen Cathedral at Sunrise," also by Monet. In yet another room Jamie recognized a portrait by Gainesborough, "Captain Thomas Matthew."

At the museum gift shop I bought stacks of photographs of various works we had seen that day to use for more bits. Then we went back to Susan's for dinner and a good night's rest before the long trip to Philadelphia the next day. Susan was accompanying us for the third time.

We spent Monday morning at the Institutes exclaiming over and over to the staff about Jamie's competence in brachiating, running, and reading. For several days he had easily been doing 30 completely independent round trips on the ladder. His hands were never sore any more. They had large rough callouses all over the palms that I filed down and wiped with alcohol every few days as instructed. He eagerly ran three miles and was never winded. And he read for enjoyment and looked intently at the bits.

Jamie was asked to sprint crawl and sprint creep up and down the hall outside one person's office, and then commended on his fine form and speed. He was even observed running a short distance outdoors. We pointed out to the people who watched him crawl, creep, and run that he had recently complained of pain in his left leg, his good leg, when he ran or did sprints. Once or twice it had been severe enough that we had to stop running or crawling, and go on to something else. Each person told us that pain was typical and to be expected, and that we should not worry about it.

They watched Jamie brachiate. Again we mentioned that Jamie frequently experienced pain, in his left shoulder this time. We wanted assurance that the constant beating the shoulder took from uneven brachiation was not causing an injury on his good side. We were given that assurance.

They watched us do a respiratory patterning on Jamie. We used our own vest on him as it was made to his measurements, and we had been told to bring it. We were asked whether we thought Jamie brachiated any better after respiratory patterning, or whether he ran any better because of it. In all honesty we had to admit that we hadn't noticed any change in his breathing. We hoped they had some way of measuring the change that we amateurs could not perceive, because we had put considerable faith in this new technique when we had first learned about it.

All in all, we had the usual number of brief interviews and measurings on this first day, interspersed with long waits in the now very familiar big waiting room. The waiting room was filled with old friends and, to our surprise, many new people. Several more members of our original class were inexplicably missing. We speculated with those present. Had the missing ones been unable to come at this time? Had they been unable to meet their goals and been obliged to postpone their third visit? Had they cured their kids? Or had they simply given up? Some of the new people were third time visitors from another class. We guessed that as classes got smaller, they were combined.

Some of the new people were not back for the third evaluation, but had been coming for many years. We talked to a mother who had been doing the program with her daughter with Down Syndrome for six years. That child ran ten miles a day, and was thin and well-developed—quite atypical for a child with Down Syndrome. But she could not yet read nor do complex math, and her articulation and her table manners were rather poor in our estimation. Another family was from France and had been coming with their son, who was now a young man in his twenties, for ten years. They could not speak English, but we heard through the grapevine that though he had been immobile and illiterate when he began, he was now athletic and read and comprehended books on nuclear physics. His only remaining problem was that he needed to learn some practical life skills—such as how to get around in his own hometown without getting lost, and to live independently.

The day's appointments were over by midafternoon. As we were leaving, we ran into a couple we knew from the start. They were distraught because they had been told to go home. In the Institutes' view, they had not worked hard enough to meet the goals that had been set for their daughter that period. They insisted that they had done their best, and had just figured that the goals were unrealistic. They were told not to come back until they met their current goals. I wondered if they would ever return.

The next two days were spent in the lecture hall. Just as before, the first session began with a staff member listing superlative achievements, determined by the previous day's interviews and evaluations. Each achievement was followed by supportive clapping from the rest of the parents. Jamie was praised an unprecedented four times—for doing the most daily brachiates, for consistently completing the most strenuous daily program, for reading above age level, and for frequently exceeding the number of daily maskings assigned. We enjoyed the limelight, but at the same time we were aware that this game was an ingenious part of their strategy to keep parents enthused, and eager to meet their goals, and to keep them coming back.

Now we sat in great anticipation of the first presentation. It turned out to be how to get a child from creeping to walking. We were disappointed. It included a practicum. All the parents put on overalls and crept, one by one, across the stage under the critical eye of the lecturer. Then we all walked across a balance beam, the purpose being to experience how unsteady a child felt when walking for the first time.

Then two new experimental devices were described. One was for children who moved their arms and legs all the time, but didn't get anywhere. It was called the Vehicle for Initial Crawling, or Vic (and the inventor's name happened to be Vic, too). The child wore a plastron, or vest-like apparatus, that contained an air disc run by a compressor. It suspended him in the air and allowed the child's random motions to result in forward movement. The device was being developed by NASA at no cost to the Institutes, we were told. The other new device, still being worked on, was akin to Chinese gloves. Their purpose would be to help a child with a poor grip to hold on to the overhead ladder.

As the two days passed, we realized that we had been spoiled by the content, delivery, and applicability of the lectures we had heard during our previous two visits to the Institutes. The content was mildly interesting this time, but not stimulating. The delivery was low-key and not dynamic because Glenn Doman was absent, busy, we were informed, working on his next book, *How to Multiply Your Baby's Intelligence*. And this time, the applicability of the various topics to our specific case was marginal.

We listened to a history of the intelligence program. They had been amazed by a parent who had taught his immobile child to read, thereby demonstrating that there was no relation between brain injury and intelligence. That had been 18 years ago, and since then every child had been put on a reading program. Then another staff member stepped up to reiterate all that we had already been taught about reading. She reemphasized that reading is a neurological function and not an academic subject, as believed by the schools. The brain, which lives in the dark, cannot tell whether language comes in via the visual or the auditory pathway because by the time it arrives it is just a chemical message transmitted through tubes. The one interesting thing that she did say was that categories of reading words should not rhyme or look alike. That is not only confusing, but boring. Bellybutton and toenail or spaghetti and liverwurst are more easily remembered and more enjoyable than sit, fit, mit, bit; and so on. Yet I had seen spelling books in the elementary schools that contained lessons with words like sheep, sweep, green, seen, or pain, main, rain, train.

Next we listened to two ladies from the Institute for the Achievement of Physiological Excellence give a rundown on every vitamin that the human body needs—why it is needed and where it can be obtained. It was a review of a college nutrition course I had taken and restated exactly what was on a chart I had hanging inside one of my kitchen cabinets. I was willing to concede that vitamins were vital to anyone's general health, but no dosage or special combination of vitamins could cure cerebral palsy, and that cure was our sole reason for coming to the Institutes.

The very last lecture on Wednesday was as boring as any I had ever attended. It concerned a matter best decided by individual families, and was delivered by a person whose lack of geniality and expression was matched only by our advocate's. The topic was The Law. The intent was to teach parents how to control and punish their children in order to get them to behave and to respect adults and do the program. She used a negative approach and spoke mostly of rules and fines. This angered several parents. We did not need to be told how to raise our children! And especially not in such a controlled atmosphere, where discussion was never permitted. We were aware that behavior modification had to be a part of some children's programs, but that should be taught only to the appropriate families, or to those who asked for help. Just imposing the program itself on Jamie had proven, to my dismay, my ability to bend, and even break, another human being. We did not need any more rigidity in our household.

Having wasted two days, we were anxious to find out on Thursday and Friday what Jamie's new program would be like.

Our first appointment was with a black-jacketed member of the Institute for the Achievement of Physical Excellence. As usual, I filled out the blanks on the blue forms as he dictated. We were to continue with four five-minute cross patterns a day. We were to discontinue marathon crawling and creeping as Jamie would only be required to do sprints. He was to slowly work up to 30 20-yard crawl sprints a day, with the goal of doing each one in less than 15 seconds. He was to slowly work up to 35 30-yard creep sprints a day, with the goal of doing each one in less than 13 seconds.

One day a week, Jamie was not to do any patterning or crawling or creeping. He was to go on a 12-mile hike in the woods. The terrain should be as difficult as possible. He should have to step over logs, slip on leaves, and duck under branches. He was to walk six miles the first time, and add one mile each week, working up to the 12 miles, with the ultimate goal of doing it in less than five hours. I knew as I wrote this that it sounded like a lot, and that there would be difficulties due to Alden's hip and the onset of winter in New England, but I didn't have time to think about it because our instructor was moving on to running.

Jamie's new running goal was to slowly increase his present three miles a day to six miles five days a week, each time in less than 65 minutes. The other two days he was to run only three miles, in less than 30 minutes, and to do 60 running sprints—20 100-yard sprints, each in less than 35 seconds, 20 80-yard sprints in less than 25 seconds each, and 20 40-yard sprints in less than ten seconds each.

As always, all creeping, crawling, and running was to be timed and recorded, and for sprints, we were to send in with our interim report the best time and the average time for each set of sprints each day.

I boldly interrupted his spiel to bring up again the matter of the mild pain Jamie had complained of several times in his lower left leg. We had hoped that since we had mentioned it on Monday an examination by the doctor on the staff might be part of Thursday's or Friday's agenda. He said that medical attention was not necessary as these types of pains worked themselves out.

Next was brachiation. Jamie would gradually increase his quota to 80 round trips a day. That was almost triple what he had been doing up to now! Half of the round trips were to be done in the usual manner, with the special goal of doing six round trips nonstop every day. But now we were to learn about two new ways to brachiate. Jamie was to do 20 round trips sideways and 20 round trips twisting. Our instructor had dismissed Jamie's leg pain so authoritatively that I didn't bother to bring up his shoulder pain. He took us downstairs to that room full of ladders to teach Jamie the two new brachiating skills.

Another staff member was sitting in the room, writing in her notebook. As she paused to watch Jamie on the ladder, she and our instructor exchanged a knowing glance and a nod. To us she said, "He's going to make it! I've never seen anyone on the program so short a time brachiate so well."

The two new ways were harder because Jamie couldn't get off his right hand so quickly when doing them. He had to support his weight longer on it. Thus he required some support at the waist from an adult to do these kinds of brachiating. The eventual goal was of course 100 percent independence for all 80 round trips. As Jamie and the instructor practiced, Jennifer observed carefully and practiced on another ladder.

We went back to the waiting room to pore over the new numbers. We had anticipated an increase, but this seemed unbelievable. How much could be fit into one day? What would they ask of us after the next visit, and the next? Where was the leveling off point?

The next day we had several brief appointments with maroon-jacketed representatives of the Institute for the Achievement of Physiological Excellence. Jamie's nutritional and vitamin supplements were to remain the same. The total number of daily maskings was to be 40, but now we were to leave the mask on each time for two minutes instead of one. And as for respiratory patterning, we were to discontinue it permanently.

My own respiration skipped a breath at this latter declaration. Hadn't Glenn Doman last time devoted almost a day of lectures to the importance of regular and deep respiration to brain injured children? How could they throw it out? They threw it out based on our own report of its questionable value. We were the judge, they said, not they.

While I was shocked at this, Alden apparently was not, for as we were being ushered out of the little room, he gallantly offered my respiratory patterning vest—"since we won't be needing it any longer"—as a contribution to the Institutes—"for those who might not be able to make their own."

' Now my respiration skipped several beats. I wanted to scream a protest to this thoughtless act of my husband! I had spent hours cutting, sewing, quilting! I wanted desperately to keep it, even if it only gathered dust in the attic with the old casts. But I couldn't interfere, as I watched the vest pass from Alden's hands to the young woman's hands, without appearing heartless and trivial. It was mine, full of my toil and Jamie's toil, but it was gone forever.

Jennifer, who had endured so much at home, had to put up with the further insult of being reprimanded this Friday afternoon by a senior staff member. We were in a hallway going to our last appointment of the week, and Jennifer, bored and tired of being quiet and patient, was understandably being sassy and resistive. The staff member, who happened to be coming out of her office, sternly told Jennifer to stop it immediately or else Mommy and Daddy would not bring her with them the next time. How dare she so insensitively threaten my daughter! How much control over our lives did these people want to exert? First the lecture on The Law and now this.

I just strolled by, clenching my teeth and dragging Jennifer. We entered the office of a camel-jacketed young woman of the Institute for the Achievement of Intellectual Excellence. Jamie and Jennifer busied themselves with some bits that were lying around. Benji crept under the table, and Alden and Susan and I sat down and braced ourselves for the expected increase in bits and words. At first it sounded as if she were actually assigning fewer words when I heard her say that Jamie must now be shown ten categories of five (instead of ten) words three times a day. But my relief was short-lived, for in her next breath she told me to retire two categories a day, instead of one. I would still need ten new word cards for each day. The only difference was that while Jamie would actually see fewer cards a day—50 a day instead of 100—each card would be active for only five days instead of ten. Jamie would have to learn them more quickly. In addition, one of the categories of five was to have a simplified dictionary definition written on the back that I would read to Jamie each time that category came up.

As for books, Jamie was to continue to read a new one a day, either homemade or commercial. It should take no more than five minutes, and we were admonished to be sure that the print was large enough and that the material was sophisticated enough.

The bits program was likewise to remain the same—ten categories of ten pictures, each pack of ten to be shown three times a day, and one pack retired and one new one added every day. She gave us one helpful suggestion for new categories. We should make accurate sketches, using an encyclopedia or other reference books as a guide, of such things as the human ear or eye, the human skeleton, machines, engines, plants, or whatever, and then Xerox many copies of each one, and on each one color in just one part so that it would stand out, and name it. That would be one bit.

And the instant math program, whose dot cards made up one category of bits, was essentially unchanged. We had on Monday expressed our doubt that Jamie was absorbing any of it, but they decided to try once more for fear of giving up too soon on what could be a useful tool to Jamie. We were to start over with presenting the equations, and we were to show him only five a day instead of ten. When we were done with the 400 equations that were already on the cards, we were to present fractional and decimal equations, which she now handed us on yellow printouts, to be copied onto the backs of my dot cards in my spare time.

There was one more element in Jamie's intelligence program. It was called programs of intelligence. I was to use my retired bits of intelligence and write one significant fact of information on the back of each one. I was to prepare five categories of five programs of intelligence, and show them three times a day, twice on the picture side while I read the program on the back, and once on the side containing the fact, which he would read silently along with me. Every day I was to retire one packet of five programs of intelligence, and add a new category of five. So now I would dust off my hundreds of used bits and delay their final deposit in the attic a while longer.

We decided to drive home on Friday afternoon again, but not before another $200 visit to the Institutes' bookstore. We bought a five-month supply of vitamins, as our next appointment wasn't until the end of March. We bought more books to cut up for bits. And we bought Jamie and Jennifer each a pair of sturdy leather hiking boots. They were a new item at the bookstore, and since nearly every family had been assigned a weekly 12-mile hike, they were selling well.

During the long hours in the car, we did our usual deciphering of the demands of the new program. Six miles of running. Twelve miles of hiking. Eighty round trip brachiates. Sixty-five crawling and creeping sprints. Sixty running sprints. Bits of intelligence. Programs of intelligence. Oh, God, I just wanted to fly to Hawaii or Guam or Africa or anywhere where they never heard of the program and where I could just be warm and let my mind go blank.

23
Questions

Are there negative consequences of the application of the method?
Cohen, Birch, & Taft, 1970, p. 309

Saturday morning I felt my life was in a state of chaos and disorder. Several half-packed suitcases lay on the bedroom floor, and beside them was a heap of dirty laundry. My kitchen counter looked like a drug store with more than two dozen little dark bottles of assorted vitamins covering it. And there were two dead goldfish in the slimy bowl on the kitchen table. Only Jello had survived the week without clean water or food.

The thought of making the materials for Jamie's huge intelligence program was overwhelming. Where could I get more bits? We had been told in August that it took between 5,000 and 10,000 bits to significantly raise a child's intelligence quotient. We had only made around 500 so far. And where was I going to get the facts to turn all those bits into programs of intelligence? How much more could I expect my friends to help me? How could such a skinny, unsteady kid run six miles, or hike 12 miles in the woods? Who wanted to do any of this with him? What would I do about Christmas? I had always had my shopping done by November in the past, and could relax and enjoy the holidays. I hadn't bought a thing. Where would I get the time or the money or the energy or the enthusiasm this year?

I had to pull myself together and face my responsibilities. I put Jamie's I'M GONNA WIN! shirt on him, and I put on my I WILL SURVIVE button. I told myself that the Institutes knew what they were doing. They had set unattainable goals for us before, and we had attained them. We would again.

On Sunday, Day 178, we officially resumed the program. Jamie was unable to do any independent brachiation. A week's rest had softened him and his hands and his shoulder hurt all over again. At the end of the day our backs ached from carrying him back and forth under the ladder.

Alden picked up a couple of topographical maps, and he decided that he and Dick would take Jamie and Jennifer on the hike every Sunday, starting today, while I stayed home with Benjiman to work on bits and programs of intelligence. It would be fun to explore the trails in the woods along the seacoast, and it would not hurt Alden's arthritic hip any more than it already hurt, he said. Yet I wondered how he could walk 12 miles on rough terrain when he could not easily walk smooth fairways and was obliged to use a golf cart? This first Sunday they estimated that they walked only three miles and it took them two hours. They would try harder the following Sunday, they promised.

I discovered, as I desperately tried to get the first five categories of five programs of intelligence ready that afternoon while they were gone, that a good source of useful information about some of my individual bits was hidden—on the backs of the bits. This was especially true of the plant cards and postcards and museum cards. I had to carefully peel the pictures away from their cardboard backings, record the facts contained thereon, and reattach the bits to the cards. From then on I never glued without first copying down vital information that might appear on the reverse.

Jennifer had no school on Monday or Tuesday, due to a teachers' workshop and Armistice Day. She wandered around like a lost soul, fighting with me every chance she got. Jamie's time was so structured and hers was so unstructured. I could only give her attention if I had a spare moment between diaper changes or brachiates or sprints. She was full of nervous energy. Her foot was tapping—no, banging—all the time. She even began to be rough with Benjiman, and I could no longer trust her with him.

Those two days were a dismal loss. Jamie's crawling and creeping sprints were extremely slow (20 to 30 seconds each). He was totally unable to do sideways or twist brachiates. Jennifer continually interrupted. I was anxious for her to be back in school the next day and for Lynne to be here in the morning to take over for an hour.

Were we back to square one? We had thought that from here on brachiating would be easy, and that Jamie's cure was in sight. Now my back and arms ached from carrying him under the ladder while his arms went through the motions but carried no weight. How much longer before his hands toughened up again to do the old kind of brachiating, and how much longer before he mastered this new kind of brachiating, so that, besides relieving my muscle strain, we could get back on the road to progress again? Or would they just think up new ways for Jamie to brachiate next time? Backwards? Upside down?

With winter coming, I had anticipated that running outdoors would eventually be impossible. The principal at Jamie's school had granted us permission to use the gym and the corridor at school for running, after school hours. A week after we got back from Philadelphia we had a snowstorm. After Alden got home from work, Jamie and I braved driving the slippery back roads to the school. While Jamie ran around and around, I carefully measured, and figured that 35 times around equalled a mile. He ran three miles in 35 minutes, a new record. That was because there were no hills, no dogs to make him turn and run the other way, no cold-induced runny nose to wipe, and no right mitten that kept falling off a limp hand. I ran a few laps, but mostly I just sat on the sidelines with my clicker. Afterwards, he did his 60 running sprints, each only a few seconds over his goal.

Later on, at home, my faithful neighbor Susan Monday walked over through the blizzard twice to cross pattern. She had magnanimously called to offer her services because she had correctly suspected that all the scheduled volunteers for the day had canceled due to the slippery roads.

The next day was sunny. Judi and Jane came over for their regular patterning time at noon. As usual, Judi brought lunch, unloaded my dishwasher, and prepared to take Jennifer home with her to play with her daughter. Alden always picked Jennifer up at Judi's on his way home from work on Wednesdays. After the second cross pattern, Jamie was doing his sprint crawls up and down the hallway. He watched wistfully as Jennifer and Judi's kids were getting into their snowsuits to go out and play at Judi's in the new snow. To top off the insult, I had let Jennifer wear Jamie's snowsuit because she had outgrown hers. How much more could he take?

That evening he ran 4 ½ miles up and down the school corridor. Nine round trips was one mile, so he made 40 ½ round trips. He weaved and limped more than usual, and he fell three times. It took him 58 minutes. He said his left leg hurt.

As the second week of the new program wore on, we were no closer to meeting any goals, neither in terms of the amount nor the time required. Jamie's running was sporadically good, but more often than not he was slowed by pain. The same was true of the 30 crawling sprints. They too hurt his lower left leg, on the shin. Creeping didn't hurt because he landed on his knee and the lower leg was free. I tried to be tough at the beginning of the week by telling him that I wouldn't count any crawl sprint that was over 25 seconds. By Friday I abandoned that rule, and we sang a new song to an old tune—Pain, Pain, Go Away. His brachiating wasn't improving either. He couldn't even do forward ones alone because of the pain in his shoulder. I kept forcing him to try because, like the hand sores that eventually became tough callouses, the shoulder pain couldn't be overcome by my bearing his weight, I told myself. He had to do it. I gave him as little support as possible and he cried in agony.

Was I doing the right thing? I had thought that the first program was difficult at the time, but now I longed for the ease of it.

Alden helped Jamie do about 15 brachiates in the morning, and Lynne did about ten with him before coming upstairs to time his 35 creep sprints. That left me with the running, the crawl sprints, the cross patterning, the Institutes' intelligence programs (which was a cinch to present, it was the preparation that was enormous), the first grade program that I was doing on my own, masking, and 25 brachiates (we were only trying to reach 50 a day, not 80 yet). I began to pile all three kids into the car and do the running at the school in the afternoon so that we could all stay together when Alden got home from work. The teachers and custodians were getting to know us, and were very curious about the program. I tried to explain, but the usual sparkle in my explanation was missing.

Since we were able to get all the program done by late afternoon, we briefly contemplated not arising at the dreadful hour of 5:30. But Jamie was an early riser by nature, and he had more gusto in the morning, which steadily waned all day. And it was pleasant to be all done before supper and enjoy a relaxed mealtime and an unstressed bedtime. We deserved that much normalcy at least. Besides, once he was actually running six miles or hiking 12 miles, and doing 80 brachiates, he would be done later than now. We had to continue to get up at 5:30 a.m.

At 5:30 I quietly removed a groggy Jamie from his bed and carried his stiff body out to the cold glass kitchen table, where everything was ready to go into action. I slapped a mask on him, started the stop watch to time it, clicked it off on the clicker, poured everyone's juice and mixed an eighth of a teaspoon of powdered vitamin C in each one, hastily chopped up an apple or an orange or a banana, took off the mask, set the timer for seven minutes, handed him his apple juice, showed him ten seconds worth of bits that I grabbed from the now totally defunct planter, unzipped his warm blue sleeper and dressed him in the clothes I had laid out the night before, popped bits of fruit into his mouth in between zipping and buttoning, put another mask on him when the timer rang, showed him the word cards with the definitions written on the backs, clicked off the mask and reset the timer, sat him in a chair to do a workbook page from one of the first grade books that Dixie had given me, heated water for Alden's coffee, measured milk and powder for hot cereal, put another mask on him at the sound of the bell, timed it and removed it, sent him to the bathroom, and, finally, piled the reset timer, the clickers, the stop watch, and the cup of coffee into Alden's hands, and sent them both downstairs. It was the same every morning.

My friends were more willing than ever to help with bits of intelligence and programs of intelligence. Jane researched the meaning of the colors and symbols on national flags. (Jamie later told me that the star on Israel's flag was the Star of Frank!) Judi researched a fact about each of the fish that I had already shown Jamie, and also about each of the Star Wars characters that I had also cut out of a poster and used as a category just for fun. Jeanne found facts to go with my bird collection, and Anita made a list of facts about the wildflowers. Someone drew clocks showing different times, someone glued real coins onto the cardboard in various combinations, someone else glued on a collection of different types of nails and screws, and someone else photocopied many copies of a schematic diagram of an automobile engine and named all the components. Many people helped me to collect the new car brochures at all the surrounding dealers, and Cora Jo, with the help of her husband, wrote a significant fact about each model. Everyone collected, cut, and glued for us, and entertained Benjiman and Jennifer while Jamie and I battled behind closed doors. I often wondered where I found such a willing group of human beings. Sometimes I thought I had to keep going just for them.

The third hike was a failure, as had been the first two. Jamie fell into two feet of water on a golf course. The dunking ruined the compass and the pedometer that Dick had bought for him. Alden and Dick brought Jamie home for a complete change of clothing and then headed courageously out again. But it was getting dark so early now that they could only stay out for another hour. They didn't bother to estimate how far they had gone, but it was certain that it was nowhere near the eight miles they should have reached by now.

It had been a bad day, starting with Alden being called into work for two hours that morning for a special problem that needed his guidance, leaving me to conduct the program on a Sunday morning, one of my days off, and finishing with a short, wet hike. But the night proved even worse. Benjiman and Susan and I went Christmas shopping while the others were hiking, and we got home very late. We managed to feed everyone and get the kids to bed, and were just setting down to relax, when Jennifer woke up complaining of a tummy ache. A few minutes later, she threw up voluminously in her bed. I removed and washed the sheets, but the mattress was too wet to remake. I moved her to Jamie's bed and put Jamie and Susan downstairs on the pull-out couch. Benjiman woke up with all the commotion, and played for an hour before settling down, but not without demanding another nursing first. At 2:00 a.m., Jennifer threw up again, and afterwards I had to resettle her in a sleeping bag. At 3:00 a.m., Jamie came upstairs to go to the bathroom, but couldn't find his way back to the stairway, and so yelled to us to turn on the light by our bed so he could see. At 3:30 the phone rang; it was one of the night shift workers at the shipyard calling the Navy's plastics expert for some advice. At 7:00 a.m., Jennifer threw up again, this time mercifully on the easy-to-clean kitchen floor.

By suppertime she was much improved. But late that night, Jamie threw up. The next morning, we commenced the program at 5:30 as usual. Jamie seemed recovered, but Alden and I felt it coming on. I ate nothing all day but had the dry heaves and was a grouch. Alden threw up as soon as he got home from work. Then we got dressed up and went to Theatre by the Sea because our tickets were for that night, and we had invited Judi and her husband as our guests. Alden took the next day off, which meant that he would be home for five days since the following two days were Thanksgiving vacation, and then it was the weekend.

One of Alden's cousins had called to invite us for Thanksgiving dinner, but we declined. My father sent us a cornucopia of fall flowers as he knew we were turning down all invitations. I did cook a turkey, but it was just another meal, and work as usual. We couldn't get into the school on holidays or weekends, so Jamie ran outdoors. The snowbanks made me nervous because they blocked our escape route if a car should swerve toward us. He wasn't used to the cold and the hills, and that, combined with his now constant pain, resulted in his slowest running time ever—4½ miles in 90 minutes.

The Sunday after Thanksgiving, Alden, Dick, and Jamie went on their fourth hike. Jennifer declared that she was never going with them again, and she stayed home with Susan, Benjiman, and me. She went Christmas shopping with us, and later made bits for her dolls while I made bits for Jamie. The hikers left at 11:00, and were not back at 4:00. Susan went home at 4:30, and I began to panic as it was almost dark. Every imaginable tragedy was running through my head. I got in the car, intending to pick them up, hoping that they had safely emerged from the cold woods, and were just hiking along the road. I got back at 5:00, ready to call the police, and they were home. They had gone seven miles in six hours. The ultimate goal was 12 miles in five hours. They had tried to speed Jamie up, and he had replied, "Hiking is walking, not running!"

That evening, before going back home, Dick changed Jello's cloudy water, as he did every weekend. The kids giggled when he picked up the wiggly orange fish in his bare hand, and dropped him into a temporary container while he scrubbed the algae out of the bowl. Jello was hearty, but the real reason he lived on was because Dick took loving care of him. "Is there no time for Jello in this household?" he asked, without expecting an answer.

The next day, Monday, December 1, was Day 200 on the program. And things were still not going well. I did not dare increase Jamie's running beyond the 4½ miles we had worked up to. He cried almost the whole 80 minutes that he ran up and down the school corridor. I was thankful that we were there late and the teachers had all gone home. The custodians were probably hiding in bewilderment in the utility room because I didn't see them. Jamie's spirits were equally terrible. What should we do? How could we go on? Wasn't it ever going to get better? What about our dreams of his cure?

On Friday I stopped Jamie after he had run for an hour because he had done only three miles, and his left shin was slightly swollen. When we all got back home, I called an orthopedic surgeon, who said he could see Jamie at 4:15 p.m. on Monday.

Over the weekend, Jamie did no running and no sprints. The swelling in his leg disappeared, so they went on their usual Sunday hike, with Jennifer, another couple, and their two young daughters. It took them four hours to do about six miles. That was the weekend they should have reached ten miles. Jamie lagged way behind and complained of pain.

On Monday, Jamie did his 35 sprint creeps and all 80 brachiates, with help, before his doctor's appointment. And of course he was cross patterned four times, masked 40 times, and shown his intelligence program. But he could not crawl or run.

The doctor inspired confidence in me. He asked the appropriate questions and got an accurate idea of Jamie's program. The left shin was badly swollen again, though Jamie hadn't run since Friday. He diagnosed it as shin splints, and was surprised that being into running so deeply I had never heard of the condition. He said it was a common runner's problem, and that some people even had to give up running because they continually developed shin splints. He said to use an ice pack on it four times a day for ten days, and if it wasn't all gone by then to call him again. He said no running or crawling or even creeping during that time. Jamie could walk though, as long as it did not hurt him.

The doctor sent us to the hospital for x-rays. He wanted to rule out the possibility of a hairline fracture of the fibula since Jamie did so much running for a six-year-old, and had recently had a change in running surface—from pavement to gym floor and carpeted cement, and had for two weeks worn poor shoes—his running sneakers had shrunk in the dryer and I had not been out with him yet to get new ones. As we came out of the hospital x-ray department, Jamie and I met our doctor coming in. He had followed us over since Jamie was his last patient of the day. He asked us to wait a minute while he went to check the results with the radiologist. He was apparently as anxious to know as we were. The films were negative and we went home.

That night Alden and I wondered why one of the lectures at the Institutes for the Achievement of Human Potential hadn't been on the dangers of running, including things to watch for and how to treat them, instead of on The Law.

We decided to put December's bill under the radio in the kitchen, and wait.

For two weeks Jamie did no physical part of the program except to brachiate 80 round trips a day. The pain in his shoulder had thankfully diminished. He was even doing some brachiating independently. And he was finishing about 2:00 p.m. My mood brightened a little. Now I could see that it would be possible to do the total program in a reasonable amount of time, when we ever got back to it. Sixty-five crawling and creeping sprints, done at required speed, and with time counted for rests in between, should only take an hour, and six miles of running should only take a bit more than an hour, eventually. That would add only two more hours onto the program we were now doing. And doing just brachiating now gave me the idea that maybe it would be better to do all of one thing at once and be done with it, instead of skipping around between brachiating and sprints as we had been doing. I was anxious to get back on the full program though, before Jamie and I got too used to this honeymoon.

Exactly two weeks after seeing the orthopedic surgeon, I cautiously resumed Jamie's physical program. He ran one mile in 12 ½ minutes, and did ten creep sprints and five crawl sprints. Nothing hurt. He did the same for two more days, and by Wednesday, Christmas Eve, the pain and the swelling were back.

Christmas Day, which we spent alone, Jamie did only 30 brachiates, primarily because of his swollen left leg. He also needed time to play with the big jeep with changeable tires that Santa had left. By midafternoon, he too was sluggish and had a temperature of 102 degrees.

I felt guilty every day that Jamie did not do a complete program. I had to write zeros in all the blanks on those blue sheets. What power the Institutes held over me! Why should I feel guilty? Jamie was in pain, he had a high temperature, and it was Christmas Day!

I was totally frustrated by the program and by the illnesses. I would have given anything to have been able to trade places with Susan that Christmas day. She got on a plane in Boston in record cold, minus 20 degrees Fahrenheit, and landed in Los Angeles, to visit her sister, in record heat, 90 degrees Fahrenheit.

Jamie wasn't able to do anything for four days. I showed his limp body bits and word cards, but doubted whether any of it penetrated his glazed look. I masked him, but his runny nose made it impossible to keep the masks fresh, and I was throwing away the smelly plastic things at a much faster rate than usual. He was a pathetic sight, lying there with his usually fluffy hair flattened against his head, breathing through the space made by his missing two front teeth.

Sunday, Dick, my father and his wife Helen, and Guilene—who was staying with Dad for a few days—came over and we had a belated Christmas celebration. We weren't able to do much program, so I had invited them. Jamie wanted to be well enough to play with Uncle Dick like old times, but he stayed put on the couch. Was it the lingering illness that immobilized him, or was it the fear of having to do the program again?

During dinner, someone asked if I had followed up on my idea of contacting newspapers about Jamie's story. I said no. Though we had not communicated to anyone else the doubt growing within us, Alden and I knew that the story was no longer a winner. Besides, instead of the one-time sensational splash in a news release I now intended to write a serious book from my notes. I was only waiting to find out the ending. I announced this over dessert and it was met with varying degrees of disbelief and jocularity.

Guilene asked, "What will you name it, 'Bondage, Pain, and Torture'?"

"How about 'Don't Tell Glenn Doman'?" This from Dick, who was spooning forbidden vanilla ice cream onto Jamie's forbidden pecan pie.

Jamie was the only one, in my opinion, who made a sensible comment. He looked straight into Jello's freshly scrubbed bowl and promised, "Jello, if some people will buy Mommy's book, we will buy you an aquarium!"

The whole following week Jamie's temperature hovered around 100 degrees. He did 30 to 40 brachiates a day. Many cross patterners had already canceled since it was school vacation week. I didn't try to get substitutes. I canceled the others so we wouldn't expose too many people to our germs. We slept late every morning and it was heaven.

I called Jamie's leg doctor to tell him that the little bit of running that he had done three days before Christmas had caused the pain and swelling to return. He said to give it a little more time.

The following Monday, January 4, we went back to getting started at 5:30. Even though we were only doing a light program (masking, patterning, bits, brachiating, and school work) I thought it best to be done early for two reasons. It was a perfect opportunity to spend the afternoon hours with Jennifer. And I needed to get back into the routine again before I got too soft.

Alden and I filled out the midterm report that was due at the Institutes. We carefully explained why Jamie had not been able to meet any of his creeping and crawling or running and hiking goals. We tried not to sound discouraged. We expected their reply would postpone our March appointment.

As I put January's bill under the radio with December's, I wondered if we would ever really go back.

Jamie did some creeping that week, but stopped due to pain. I called his doctor again to be sure that it was okay to be taking so long for shin splints to completely clear up. He said it could possibly take many weeks longer, and that he needed another set of X-rays to be sure there wasn't a hairline fracture.

I couldn't stand this much longer. Both the program and our health had fallen apart.

One thought that had kept me going for many months was that our 52 hostages in Iran had been confined longer than I had. Their lives and mine had come to a virtual standstill. Though I imagined myself like the hostages in some ways, I was ever mindful of one staggering difference: my confinement was entirely voluntary, nonhumiliating, and nonbrutal.

On Tuesday, January 20, 1981, as Ronald Reagan was being sworn in as the 40th President of the United States, the hostages were released. My imaginary comradeship was over. It had been 444 days for them, and it was only Day 252 for me.

How much longer before I too would be free?

The expected letter from our advocate at the Institutes arrived the following Saturday, January 24.

Dear Mr. and Mrs. Bratt,

Thank you for your Interim Report. As of the date you receive this note, please discontinue all physical programming for two weeks, except brachiation. Cut brachiation in half and do no more than one round trip at a time. During this time double your intelligence program, patterning and masking. After two weeks, begin walking every day with Jamieson, building up to 12 miles a day. The following weeks begin back on the crawling and creeping, continue with walking every day. All walking is to be done on grass or dirt only. At the end of this two week period, please call me.

All else looks good. My best to everyone.

This letter astounded me! The last time Jamie had run was Christmas Eve—exactly one month before we received this note—and even that running had already been after a two-week layoff. Did they think we were waiting with bated breath for their permission to stop a child in pain from running?

Double the intelligence program? I was already at the limit of my creativity and time for making bits. Wouldn't reading the encyclopedia accomplish the same thing?

Double the patterning? How could I get more volunteers again? Two had even regretfully resigned lately. And hadn't the Institutes assigned us only four patternings a day because they felt that was all that he needed now? Were they assigning us more just to fill up our time? And more masking for the same reason?

The most incredible part was a 12-mile daily hike on grass or dirt only! Didn't they know that it was winter in Maine? All we had was ice and snow and salted pavement. What were we to think? What were we to do?

24
The Crash of '81

Information which does not result in performance is useless.
                        LeWinn, et al., 1966, p. 52

That letter had a profound effect on us. We shared its contents with Susan and Dick when they arrived. We had all had varying degrees of doubt, either voiced or unvoiced, at different times, but now it had come to a boiling point. We had to decide whether or not to go on with the Institutes' program.

I was not a quitter. I was committed to a two-year program at the Institutes for the Achievement of Human Potential, and I felt it was my duty to Jamie and to myself to complete it.

In other situations, completion gave me a peaceful feeling of gaining something. But now, I asked myself, what would I gain, besides exhaustion and bad memories, by completing the Institutes' program?

It boiled down to two questions. Were there any real changes in Jamie that could honestly be attributed to the program? And could we realistically hope for any further changes in continuing the program? The four of us discussed these questions for many hours Saturday night.

Over Sunday morning brunch, Susan told of the dream she had the night before. She had been at the Institutes with us. She knew they wanted to be rid of her because she was a negative influence on us. All she ever did was eat their food and never paid them any money. One of the lectures was at the seashore where they were talking about lung development and demonstrating it by comparing it to gill development. While out on a boat, someone who knew Susan feared water and couldn't swim "accidentally" pushed her overboard. She struggled and somehow managed to make it back to shore, and the staff pretended to be glad. Later in the dream, she was driving to the Institutes and was stopped by the police and arrested for insubordination when she had accidentally touched her horn. The police had been paid by the Institutes to arrest her. This dream told me that Susan, too, was struggling with her own guilt about betraying the faith she had once had in the Institutes.

The next evening, when Alden and I were alone, we continued our conversations. We found that our topics fell into three broad categories: the effect of the program on our personal lives, the personalities and policies of the people who had assigned the program to us, and the different aspects of the program itself.

First, we looked at the ways the program had upset us at home. We had moved furniture and destroyed grass and put toys in the attic. We had lost contact with many friends, we had lost sleep, we had lost money and valuables, we had lost vacation time, we had imposed on volunteers. We had lost precious time with Benjiman, Jennifer, and with each other. Maybe we had even lost time with Jamie even though we had spent so many hours with him.

We had a strange order of priorities. We were governed by a force outside our home. I forced all three of my children to submit to demands that I myself wasn't always sure of, and I did it so well that I was sometimes ashamed of my behavior.

But whereas I understood my bizarre behavior, and could alter it at any time, and indeed longed to be free of the force that was driving me, what about Jennifer? A psychologist would have a field day dissecting her behavior! She had recently instructed us to call her Angela, and had even written that name on her school papers. When I mistakenly addressed her as "Jennifer," she made a name tag that said "Angela" and pinned it to her dress. Did she want to be someone else, someone who did not have to deal with the program? Some days she begged me to play baby with her. She wrapped herself in a blanket, sucked her thumb, and demanded that I cradle her. Did she want to go back to a time before the program? She twisted the right arm or the right leg off of most of her Barbie dolls, and then asked me one day if Jamie didn't have any righty, would he still have to brachiate and crawl? One day she dressed Benjiman up in a dress and put pink barrettes in his hair. Did she think that if he were a girl that might save him some day having to do the program like his older brother?

And God only knew what was going on in Jamie's mind. My constant fear was whether he hated me. Alden's constant fear was whether we were ruining his left side while trying to improve his right side. We had always maintained that one of the attractions of the Institutes' program was that, unlike the surgeries that doctors had recommended for cerebral palsy, nothing that the Institutes required could hurt Jamie. And now he was hurting. Probably psychologically and definitely physically.

Next, we vented some of the resentments we felt every time we set foot on the Institutes' grounds. They had not informed us ahead of time of the exorbitant cost, they had not been helpful when we tried to get insurance coverage, they had not arranged for Jamie to see a doctor when we complained of his pain, they had not included a lecture on shin splints, they wielded such physical and psychological control over us during the lectures, they had canceled what was supposed to be a revolutionary new technique, they had refused to give us names and addresses of children just like Jamie who had been totally cured though they assured us that there were several, they didn't supply us with ready-made bits or even supply precut cardboard, they were so disorganized that parents routinely wasted many hours or even days in Philadelphia, they assigned new programs or more programs arbitrarily just to fill up the hours of the day, and they made unrealistic demands (to hike on grass or dirt in January in Maine).

Glenn Doman, who professed to love children, never once walked through the full waiting room while we were there. In our experience, impersonality and coldness permeated the place. It was common for a staff member to poke his or her head into the waiting area and yell "Bratt" without looking up from the folder in his or her hand and then turn and walk abruptly away, expecting the eager parents to have gathered up children and belongings at a moment's notice and be following obediently behind. Very few tried to gain any sort of rapport with Jamie.

There was a constant authoritative attitude, as though they were waiting for a chance to disapprove. When I mentioned that I no longer ran with Jamie, but rather biked beside him, the revelation had been met with raised eyebrows and "Someone should run with him!" The staff member who had reprimanded Jennifer had seemed smug afterwards, like a police officer who had filled his quota of speeding tickets. We had even heard via the grapevine that one family had been told by a particularly austere member of the staff to smile more often and to act more enthusiastic or they would be kicked out.

Finally, we dared to pick apart the program itself. We felt most positive about the reading. Jamie had learned to read very well while on the program. It was partially due to their flash card method, but more due to my having written hundreds of sentences all over the wall. And now that he had arrived, was it necessary to continue teaching him by using flash cards? And he had definitely increased his general knowledge through the bits of intelligence cards. But was this the best way to go on? It seemed redundant and excessive. Who cared if Jamie knew 500 species of African wildlife or 100 varieties of antique cars or all of Michelangelo's paintings? What good did all of that knowledge do if one is in bondage due to the rigid, unyielding confines of the daily program?

We felt the least positive about the creeping and crawling and cross patterning. Were they really "closed brain surgery"? There were no tangible results other than the fact that Jamie could creep and crawl a certain distance at a certain speed. What did it have to do with curing cerebral palsy? Why had we jumped up and down and considered it to be such a milestone when he had first crept two miles? And why had we believed that crawling and creeping could uncross Jennifer's eye when Glenn Doman himself wore glasses! Creeping and crawling and cross patterning were the easiest to dismiss from our minds as we had never felt totally confident in their value from the beginning.

What about masking? Since we had been masking him, Jamie hadn't had any seizures, and his chest size had increased. Those were both goals of masking, but how could we tell if they would have happened anyway? Jamie had been seizure-free, without medication, for four months prior to his being masked daily, and his chest circumference, like any child's, had increased at varying rates since birth.

Running. Until shin splints we had run three or more miles a day at a respectable pace. But anyone reasonably mobile could accomplish that. Besides being a boost for his ego and healthy for his heart and habit-forming for future exercise, what did it do toward curing cerebral palsy? He ran flat-footed and with a limp and he would always run flat-footed and with a limp. And he would always walk flat-footed and with a limp. This in particular was a painful realization, as was this whole discussion, and my eyes brimmed with tears when I admitted it.

Next, brachiation. We were appalled to uncover similar doubts about what we had considered to be the most viable part of the physical program. Jamie had mastered 30 round trips a day, and we could probably toughen him up to reach the 80 a day they now wanted. But though we were still in awe of the fact that his weak, bent little hand could actually hold onto the rungs, it only did so for a split second. There was no corresponding improvement in how he carried that hand when he walked or in his fine motor control. He could not use his fingers to pick up anything smaller or larger than one of the rungs of the ladder. If he did manage to grab something with that hand, he would lose his grip almost immediately. We were certain that Jamie would never use that right hand to properly manipulate a pencil or a fork. It seemed then that brachiating too did nothing toward curing cerebral palsy.

Brachiating, like running, was just a sport that a mildly impaired individual could be successful at and receive praise for. This too was a courageous and painful admission. I slid off the couch and onto the floor. I buried my face in the cushion I had just been sitting on, and wet it with tears.

Oh, God, not brachiating too! I had been so sure that that had been the key! Now running was a farce and so was the brachiating. It wasn't the lost time and wasted effort that crumpled me so much as the lost hope for my Jamie. We were supposed to win! What had happened to change everything? Glenn Doman had said that children never failed, only parents failed. Had we failed?

I tried to control my desolation, and sat up against the couch, hugging my knees, Alden's strong hand on my shoulder. He was telling me, in a low voice fraught with defeat, that we had done our very best with what we had been given.

In the depths of our souls, beneath the veneer of far-fetched promises and unrealistic hopes, lay the truth. The program did not work for Jamie. Jamie would not be cured by the program. Jamie would not be cured, period.

The billboard was right. Cerebral palsy could not magically disappear. Birth defects are forever.

If I had thought the emotional crash of 1979, when Alden had cried at Jamie's bedside, had been devastating, I knew now that it had been mild compared to the rock bottom we had just hit.

PART III

AFTER THE PROGRAM

25
Letting Go

Furthermore, there is little or no evidence that any specific kind of replacement stimulation results in the rectification of the neurological defects once they have occurred.

Cohen, Birch, & Taft, 1970, pp. 309-310

The next few days and even weeks were difficult. We went on with the program as before because we did not want to give up any part of it until we were absolutely sure that it had no redeeming value. And we did not want anyone to think that we were giving up without a lot of thought. We were the ones who had convinced them that what we were doing was right. Now we had to reverse that without appearing foolish.

I began to hint to our volunteers that we might not return to Philadelphia, due to the expense, so I said, and that we might not need cross patterners much longer, since the Institutes was probably going to eliminate that anyway at our next visit. White lies were better than naked truths at this point, for them and for us. This way our patterners, who had given so much, could have time to get used to the idea, instead of feeling abruptly and ungratefully cast aside.

Besides masking, bits, and patterning, Jamie did 80 brachiates, 35 sprint creeps, and went on a walk every day. Jamie and Alden did only brachiating and masking together now in the morning since respiratory patterning and long distance creeping around the patterning table had been eliminated. When Lynne arrived, she too did just brachiation and masking with Jamie. That left me to complete about 30 to 40 brachiates with him, his 35 creeping sprints, his reading and bits and other school work, his masking, and our daily walk. No running and no crawling.

Jamie's shoulder was hurting less and he was beginning to do some brachiating independently again. We could foresee that he someday could do the whole 80 alone and we intended to work toward that. But we no longer had illusions about it curing his hand. We continued it as a good exercise for straightening his arm and preventing the withering of unused muscles. It seemed as good as any activity previously encouraged by physical and occupational therapists.

Crawling still hurt his recovering leg, so he did only creeping, which did not hurt. Though we questioned crawling and creeping, we hung on to sprint creeping while we decided what to do about it. We were on a train and it was hard to get off.

As for running, we felt that it would be a good exercise to resume in the spring, when we would be sure that his shin splints had plenty of time to heal. As with brachiating, we no longer had any dreams that running would in any way cure cerebral palsy, but it was a good exercise for a person who had limited choices for competence in sports. Running might even eventually serve as a boost to his ego by providing the opportunity to win in competition.

Until spring, when Jamie's leg and Maine roads were suitable for running, we were in fact following the suggestion of the Institutes to take a daily hike. But not 12 miles and not on grass or dirt! We walked three to six miles, on pavement. And we did it for fun and fresh air, not to "organize his cortex," as we had been told the primary goal of running was. The kids and I suited up in snow pants and down mittens every afternoon after Jamie's other work was done and Jennifer was home from school. Benjiman finally experienced the pleasure of riding on my back in the backpack, as had his sister and his brother before him. He giggled and babbled with glee, he pulled my hat off, and his nose ran incessantly. Jennifer brought along a paper bag to collect rocks and ice and other trivia. Jamie talked continually of the possibility of making it to the drawbridge and of what oil tankers and lobster boats we might see. Or the greatest thrill—what if the bridge was up?

On weekends we all went on long hikes in the York woods and along the shore. Neither Benjiman nor I had ever accompanied Alden, Dick, Jamie, and Jennifer on their former Sunday hikes. Now that the pressure of a required distance and time had dissipated, I relaxed and looked forward to this family event. My hatred of winter relented slightly as I gazed at the beauty of Maine in its frozen state.

The fresh air was invigorating, and after a few weeks it helped to begin to clear my mind of doubt and guilt about not doing the program in the exact prescribed way. If I could get over that, then I would only have to face the fact that Jamie was not cured of cerebral palsy and never would be. That was a much heavier weight to get out from under.

I stopped making new bits in February. I continued to write programs on the backs of the retried bits, and I figured that I might as well continue showing those, which I estimated would last until mid-May. I stopped making word cards and definition cards and homemade books, too. I threw away the letter cards we had used for spelling. I put the dot cards and the unused list of fraction and decimal equations in the attic. Jamie instead read commercial books and worked in his first grade math workbook every day. Since I no longer had piles of cut cardboard lined up on the planter between the living room and the kitchen, I bought 15 philodendron plants and planted them in the barren soil, hoping that they would not take too long to cascade down over the brick wall as had their predecessors.

Alden and I couldn't believe that we suddenly had nothing to do in the evenings. I read novels and Alden read the newspaper. We got to know each other again. We went out to the movies alone together for the first time in over a year. Another time we went dancing. I had forgotten that people did such enjoyable things.

Jamie and Jennifer also benefitted from the unaccustomed free time. Since Jamie was definitely going back to school in the fall, he needed to become friendly with his classmates. We found ways for this to happen. Jennifer had long wanted ballet lessons, clogs, and pierced ears like the other little girls in kindergarten. I now took the time to have these happen for her.

We were putting off writing a letter of resignation to the Institutes. We wanted to live with our decision for a while before making it official. We had to be sure that our withdrawal was not based on poverty, illness, selfishness, or laziness. And we knew that no matter what we said or how we said it, in the Institutes' view we would be failures. They would say we didn't do the program long enough or hard enough, and that we would never know what would have happened if we had done it longer and harder. Alden and I were still struggling with our private feelings of failure and guilt, and were only able to slowly give up principles and techniques we had once clung to. What had been accepted as gospel truth was not easily rejected, even in the face of new evidence. I could not write the letter of resignation yet.

At the end of February we decided not to do the program on weekends any more. It wasn't actually as abrupt as that—we had been getting more lax on weekends for some time. Jamie was ecstatic. Now he led a normal life two days out of seven. How wonderful it was for Alden and me to stay in bed another two hours.

Also in February I devised a two-part plan to gracefully eliminate the rest of Jamie's creeping and at the same time to encourage him to brachiate independently. First, I threw out all twisting and sideways brachiating because they were too difficult. They only slowed him up and discouraged him. We would work toward 80 regular brachiates. Secondly, I told him that for every round trip brachiate he did without anyone touching him, I would first throw out his 30 sprint crawls, two at a time, and then his 35 sprint creeps, one at a time. That meant that if he did 15 independent brachiates, he did not have to crawl, and if he did 35 more independent brachiates, he did not have to creep. Since he was already back to doing 30 alone, that justified to him why we already had given up all of the crawling for good, and some of the creeping. To be totally done with the creeping he needed only to increase his independent brachiates by 20. I don't know why I felt the need to make a game of it instead of just dropping it. It just felt better that way. It was taking a long time to return to normalcy.

We reached one more landmark decision in February. Starting in March, we would begin to phase out cross patterning. I made a schedule that gradually eliminated people and patterns throughout the month, and informed everyone. The final cross pattern would be done on April Fools' Day.

At last we felt ready to write the letter of resignation to the Institutes. We felt secure in our decisions. In the letter we stated two superficial reasons for our withdrawal, expenses and shin splints, and did not harangue about our innermost opinions. We expressed gratitude for Jamie's reading ability, and his freedom from seizure medication, braces, casts, and splints. We ended with mention of the fact that we intended to continue some of the program on our own. We wanted to say that we were phasing out patterning, crawling, creeping, and bits, and phasing in skating, biking, swimming, golfing. But we didn't.

I put the letter in my mailbox with confidence and a clear conscience.

26
Accept Them, And All Else

Through Todd our family learned understanding and patience. And, in a deeper sense, we learned love. For in the untouched innocence of this child, we were reminded innocence dwells in every human being.

Melton, 1986, p. 154

We received four separate letters from the Institutes in early March. One was an unsigned impersonal reply to our letter, perfunctorily wishing us luck. One was the usual monthly bill for $250. One was a form letter to all delinquent Institutes participants from Glenn Doman pleading for unpaid bills to be paid. And the fourth was a letter from their auditor, asking for confirmation of the fact that we owed the Institutes for three months, totaling $750. I found it curious that it arrived in one of the Institutes' business envelopes, imprinted with the Institutes' address and logo. Was this really an attempt on the Institutes' part to get us to sign that we were responsible for that amount and then they could legally hold us to it? We had paid November's installment during our last visit to Philadelphia, and as we had received no services since then, and did not plan to ever return, we felt we were not obligated to pay the December, January, and February bills. I wrote that explanation on the "auditor's" statement and we never got another bill from the Institutes.

I seldom watched television, even before the program, but on March 16, as I was sitting moodily alone downstairs, I turned on the TV and unexpectedly tuned in to two shows that had a profound effect on me. The first was Phil Donahue talking to children who had or used to have life-threatening illnesses, and the second was the old movie Madame X. I bawled through both heartrending shows. But they had an extra impact on me because I was struck by the fact that in both shows the mothers of those children had more to grieve about than I did. Their children were either dying or being taken away from them. These things were not happening to me—Jamie was healthy and he was with me.

I suddenly realized that I hadn't been appreciative enough of those blessings. My mind of late had been too full of grief over what Jamie could have been, not what he was. He had become "my son with cerebral palsy," not "my son with blueberry eyes." I thought about this injustice to Jamie and the resulting strain on our relationship. The two television shows were over and I was sitting quietly in the big brown recliner. I reached over to the book-shelf and found my copy of *Overload*, the most recent novel by one my favorite authors, Arthur Hailey. I had read it before the program. I remembered a poem in it I wanted to reread.

> Yes!—the "if onlys" do persist forever
> As hovering, wraithlike, used-up wishes,
> Their afterburners spent!
> "If only" this or that
> On such and such a day
> Had varied by an hour or an inch;
> Or something neglected had been done
> Or something done had been neglected!
> Then "perhaps" the other might have been,
> And other others...to infinity.
> For "perhaps" and "if only" are first cousins
> Addicted to survival in our minds
> Accept them,
> And all else (p. 152).

Before, when I had read this poem, it had only served to remind me of my guilt and heartbreak and everyday struggle. It had reinforced my determination to try to recapture what might have been. I didn't even see the last two lines then. "Accept them, And all else." That was the key to untying the knot in my soul.

I decided right then to stop dwelling on the "if onlys" and "what ifs." I was not responsible for Jamie's disability, the doctors were not responsible, and Jamie certainly wasn't responsible. I did not have the cure, the doctors did not have the cure, and the Institutes did not have the cure. What was, was. The presence of a disability should no more characterize a person than should crooked teeth or frizzy hair or fat ankles. Jamie was Jamie and I loved him no matter what.

I also reached for my copy of *Son-Rise*, written by Barry Neil Kaufman about his son Raun who had autism. I thumbed through it, reviewing his philosophy, called the Option Method, and remembering how it had helped them through despair over their son's difference. The central tenet of this philosophy was, "To love is to be happy with." Why hadn't I applied that to our situation before? Jamie was Jamie and I loved him no matter what.

I went to bed red-eyed, but with the weight of Jamie's cerebral palsy beginning to lift.

27
On Our Own Again

Are the results reported as deriving from the method directly dependent on it, or are they serendipitous consequences deriving inadvertently from the maturation of the child, the amount of time and training devoted to his care, the structuring of patterns of parental behavior, or the placebo effect of rearoused hopes for progress and improvement in functioning?

Cohen, Birch, & Taft, 1970, p. 305

St. Patrick's Day came and we were reminded that exactly a year ago our first cross patterners had come into our home and we had started our daily program. My notebook said it was only Day 308, but that was because I had considered May 1 as the official starting date, after receiving and organizing the genuine program from our first visit to the Institutes. Also I had not counted the days spent at the Institutes during the subsequent two visits. I decided to stop counting. What did it matter how many days? Timing and counting were not so desperately important to us any more.

Jamie's seventh birthday fell on a Saturday. We went to Jennifer's ballet show in the morning. At noon Dick arrived with a new fishing rod for Jamie. After just a little practice Jamie was proud to show us that he could wind up the reel with his right hand just fine. In the late afternoon, we took Jamie and his friends bowling, a great one-handed sport we discovered, and then out to Papa Gino's for pizza. He made his own pizza in the kitchen as he had done the previous year, and afterwards I served his sailboat cake.

Soon Jamie would be doing only a three-part program—masking, brachiating, and running. We were hanging onto masking in case it was in fact preventing seizures. Independent brachiating was slowly improving. And we resumed running on the last day of March. It took the place of our daily walk. I planned to work very gradually up to three miles (not six) and I wasn't going to pressure him to break any speed records. I bought a secondhand bicycle baby seat for Benjiman since it would be necessary that he accompany me on Jamie's runs because the last day that I would ever have volunteers in the house to babysit was fast approaching.

On Wednesday, April 1, Judi, Jane, and I did the last two cross patterns on Jamie. After lunch we celebrated by devouring most of the ice cream and cream puff pie that Judi brought. We were having a party the next Saturday night for all our patterners and their husbands. Early in the week, I began to prepare every fancy hors d'oeuvre and dessert I could think of, and Alden's music group, composed of himself and two other shipyard workers who called themselves "The Yardbirds," rehearsed for the event. As a gift for each friend, I bought a large quantity of neck scarves of assorted colors, and hired an artist to silk screen the Institutes' logo on the corner of each scarf.

The party was a great success. Everyone conversed, ate and listened to music. Most of the people knew each other. I passed out the scarves and thanked each one as she left.

Our new version of the program was as follows:

5:30-6:00	wake up, dressed, masking, fruit and juice, bits
6:00-7:15	30 brachiates with Alden, masking, bits
7:15-7:55	3 workbook pages, more breakfast, masking
7:55-8:10	outdoor break
8:10-9 or 10	brachiates with Lynne
9 or 10-10:45	reading and other school work, snack
10:45-11:30	run
11:30-12:00	play outside with Jennifer
12:00-12:30	lunch
12:30-2:00	finish brachiates and bits.

Even this modified version of the Institutes program took a big chunk out of the day. We still got up at 5:30 because I needed Alden to be responsible for part of the program and because with summer coming I wanted to be done early enough in the afternoon so that we could have some pool or beach time. Masking, bits, and school work took only a minimum amount of time and effort, and the latter two would soon be phased out completely. Crawling and creeping were already phased out because he was doing at least 50 brachiates alone. That left brachiating and running as the major aspects of Jamie's therapy.

Jamie's running and brachiating continued to improve. Soon he reached his goal of three miles and 80 brachiates. I was sometimes curious to know what the exact number of total miles was that Jamie had run, or crawled or crept in the past year, or the total distance he had brachiated. But I just didn't seem to have the energy or the inclination to flip through the records and figure it out. I wasn't going to brag about it to anyone.

28

Grade Placement

The Institutes' goal for every child on their program is to eventually enroll him in a regular class with children his own age.

Melton, 1971, p. 192

The principal at Jamie's school called to remind us that there had to be a Pupil Evaluation Team meeting (PET) before the end of the school year to discuss Jamie's progress and his reentry into the public schools. Before the meeting she wanted Jamie tested.

On Wednesday, May 13, we discussed Jamie's performance on those tests. His reading, word recognition, comprehension, and general knowledge all showed ability at or above second grade level. His math and spelling scores on the achievement tests were considerably lower—at the early first grade level. I was surprised at the low math score, since I considered that to be one of Jamie's strengths, along with reading. The examiner said that the score could be falsely low because he gave the math part of the achievement test first, and perhaps Jamie had not yet warmed up to him or to the testing situation. The principal disputed this, saying she felt Jamie didn't really comprehend numbers. I replied that I believed that he knew not only "fiveness" but "eightyness" as well. He didn't simply read 80 in a book, he experienced it every day and he understood exactly its enormity. I explained that he learned place value from rocks lined up on the crawl course in groups that represented the tens and ones. I explained that 22 times around the kitchen table had been to him "10 and 10 and 2." They looked at me like I was from outer space. How could I expect them to understand the relation of rocks on a crawl course to figures and computations? Or that tough calluses on the palms of his hands were proof of his conquest of large numbers?

I left without further dispute. I never doubted Jamie's academic readiness for second grade. But now I felt certain that we were going to run into opposition at the upcoming PET meeting, only two weeks away. As soon as I got home I called Dixie and Susan. They didn't underestimate Jamie's ability. They were objective, credible professionals who would support our viewpoint. I wanted them at that PET meeting.

A few days later, when Jamie was running his three miles, we went by a house where a young boy was playing with the *Star Wars* spaceship known as the Millennium Falcon. Jamie eyed it covetously. With renewed determination, he set out to earn this toy which I had promised to buy for him when he completed all brachiates without support for five consecutive days. For the next five days he screamed at me if I came anywhere near him while he brachiated for fear that I would touch him and thus invalidate his accomplishment. His hands were raw and bleeding from the sudden, continued increase. I bandaged and taped them, but that didn't eliminate the pain. He winced and bit his lip as he went from rung to rung. He did it, and I was mightily proud of him as I took him to the department store. He did 80 every day from then on.

Jamie ran exceptionally well, and without pain, now that he had met his three mile goal. One hot spring day, Judi and her kids were over for an early season swim, and Judi, who jogged occasionally, offered to run with Jamie while I relaxed with the kids around the pool. "I'll just run zigzag if he lags," she boasted. Three miles and 35 minutes later, Jamie came running down the driveway, kicked off his shoes, and jumped into the water, totally non-winded as usual. Two minutes later Judi came down the hill, red-cheeked and puffing. Jamie had been ahead the whole time. At the two dead ends where he reversed, she had turned around at the same time as he did even though she was several yards behind him. But Jamie always caught up and passed her. "He never slowed down, not even on hills," Judi complained. And she never had to zigzag.

We had the meeting to settle the matter of Jamie's reentry into public school on May 27. There were nine people present and it lasted almost two hours—both unusual facts for a PET meeting. At the principal's request, Alden and I opened the discussion by giving a brief and positive description of the program Jamie had been on and the physical and academic progress we felt he had made. Lynne, a daily observer and a participant from the school, confirmed our statement.

The principal and the male examiner followed this with a report of Jamie's recent math testing scores and, on the basis of those, made the suggestion that first grade would be the appropriate grade placement for Jamie. We had expected this and we had our defense ready. We expressed our belief, supported by Susan and Dixie, both teachers, that the math score was simply an inaccurate reflection of his actual understanding. We pointed out too that Jamie's reading score was almost at the third grade level. The opposition countered with, "Handicapped children always pick something to excel in."

"But reading is the best predictor of intelligence, not math," offered Susan.

Two other reasons for retention were then brought up. Jamie was small for his age, and Jamie had been removed from the school routine for a year and would therefore need an easy year academically to readjust. My response was that being small was an advantage only if one had to stay back, but definitely not a reason in itself for retention. I tried to explain why Jamie's readjustment to school would be a breeze for him. Nothing could match the intensity of the program he had endured for the past year. But that was almost impossible to convey. They feared he would tire easily, and that he might have a separation problem from me.

Another objection was brought up by the two negative members of the team. Creating success was the most important goal, and Jamie would find the work in first grade easier, they said. Well of course he would! He had already done first grade work, and done it well. What a blow to sit down at his desk, open up the same books and do the same work all over again. He would feel like a failure, I contended, not a success. A child who had faced failure all his life, whether playing baseball or zipping his pants, didn't need to be faced with it again.

Then we were vehemently told that the feeling of failure at retention was instilled by parents. We disagreed. Except in cases where parents were excessively punitive for poor grades, the child's peers did a magnificent job of excluding a child they felt didn't measure up. Jamie knew the normal progression of grades. Jamie also knew he was a year older than his sister and therefore ahead of her in school, and Jennifer knew she should be behind her brother in school. Psychologically, for both, it would be better for Jamie to be at the bottom of the heap in the second grade than at the top of the heap in the first grade. If ever it was necessary for any of our children to repeat a grade, we would then deal as best we could with the resulting emotional and social problems. But we should not now have to cope with Jamie's further feeling of failure since it was not academically necessary for Jamie to repeat a grade at this time.

We knew that legally the parents had the final say. Alden finally said, "Look, we've hashed this over enough. Berneen and I, as the ones who know Jamie the best, have already decided that we want Jamie in the second grade in the fall, despite any opinions to the contrary. We'll take the responsibility for the placement."

"Write that down!" shot the principal to the person who was taking minutes of the meeting for Jamie's permanent record. There followed an abbreviated discussion of teacher selection and whether the aide would still be needed. We felt the teacher should not be a right-by-the-book type. A stickler for penmanship would doom Jamie. Yet we didn't want a teacher to mollycoddle Jamie because he was different. We just needed one who would allow some variation when needed, who would be willing to keep close contact with me so I could help Jamie at home when needed. Such a teacher was chosen.

The school wanted to dispense with the financial burden of an aide. Perhaps that was even an underlying reason for their attempt to keep Jamie in first grade—he might get along without an aide there. But we insisted that the presence of an aide was crucial to his performance, no matter what grade he was in. Jamie needed individualized oral repetition of instructions, he needed to be prodded to complete an assignment, he needed help in finding his place on a page, he needed help remembering where he put something yesterday or a minute ago, and his spatial orientation in the room or in the whole school was apt to be confused.

I foresaw other responsibilities for an aide. Jamie frequently came out of the bathroom undone, his chin was usually covered with food after a meal, he drooled occasionally, and he had a new habit of chewing vigorously on his cuff or collar. None of these characteristics brought peer admiration. Alertness and discretion on the part of the aide would be invaluable.

Also, there was a safety factor. Jamie might step out onto the parking lot in front of a car, get stranded on the jungle gym, or knocked over in the dismissal rush. Besides, another child with cerebral palsy, a little girl Jamie knew from kindergarten and his rehab days, would be in his class and could use help in the classroom as she was not quite walking alone yet. It was agreed that an aide for Jamie should be included in the budget, though we were warned it would only be for half a day. And, to our dismay, Lynne was getting a full-time, higher-paying job and would not be available. We would have to settle for an unknown aide.

I was never one to wish the summer away before it had even started, but with the issue of his grade placement settled, I began looking forward to eliminating further program components and a new beginning at school for Jamie.

29
Back to School

When I got away from it, it was such a relief.
Parent quoted in Warshaw, 1982, p. 184

Susan and Dick continued to come to Kittery most weekends, even though we hadn't needed them for help with the program since February. They both admitted they now looked forward to the weekends with us instead of dreading them. It had been a true test of friendship.

At the end of August we decided we would no longer get up at 5:30 a.m. It was beginning to be dark and dismal at that hour. We just couldn't take it any longer. We were burned out and had no more energy or drive. Soon Jamie would be in school anyway, and he would be better off to go each morning fresh and happy than tired and resentful from two hours of early morning programming. Until school started, we would do what we could during normal daylight hours, and then do brachiating, running, and masking after school to maintain his body strength and tone.

Dick was as excited as any of us about Jamie's imminent return to school. He also put Jamie in charge of changing Jello's water once a week. He thought that the logical sequence of steps required to do this would help Jamie organize his approach to lessons in school.

First, it was necessary to fill a small plastic container with clean water, then pour the dirty water from the glass fish bowl through a strainer so that Jello would land in the strainer and not go down the drain with the water, then gently dump Jello from the strainer into the clean water in the plastic container, then scrub and rinse the slimy algae from the glass bowl and the ceramic castle, refill that bowl with fresh water, and then finally pour the clean water and Jello from the plastic container into the large freshly-scrubbed glass bowl.

It was nerve-racking but interesting to watch Jamie try to remember these steps. The whole scenario, repeated exactly the same way time after time with no improvement, illustrated Jamie's approach to life in general. He was mildly confused, disorganized and disoriented, even in familiar surroundings. His actions were a series of delayed responses.

To change Jello's water, Jamie first stood on a chair at the sink. When he realized he didn't have all his equipment handy, he got down and got the empty plastic container. Then he knew he needed the strainer, but it always took him a few seconds to recall which cupboard I kept it in, though I always kept it in exactly the same place. Ready again, he climbed up on his chair. Next, he put some water in the plastic container. Jennifer, always close by, checked to be sure it wasn't hot. Jamie then lifted up Jello's bowl shakily with one hand and started to dump it into the small container of clean water. At the last moment it dawned on him that it would mix dirty water with clean water, and that the small container would overflow. So he would put Jello's bowl down and instead try to fit the strainer in the small opening at the top to capture Jello. It wouldn't fit but he kept trying anyway. Finally, he put the strainer on the counter and was ready to pour. Once again he picked up Jello's bowl and again he put it down when he saw that the strainer really should be down in the sink, rather than on the counter. That taken care of, he then dumped, jerkily, while Jennifer turned away, praying that his aim would be accurate. When Jello, usually followed by the ceramic yellow and orange castle, landed in the strainer, Jamie stopped pouring after a second or two, put down the bowl with incredible slowness, looked absentmindedly for a place to put the castle, and finally picked up the strainer and safely deposited a gasping Jello in the container of clean water. Jennifer breathed a sigh of relief.

Sometimes Dick or I led Jamie through these steps with questions to sharpen his observation, but most often we just let him stumble through it. Dick once said, "The world will little note nor long remember what poor Jello had to endure for the sake of educating his keeper."

Tuesday, September 8, was the first day of school. For the third year in a row I wept when the bus came. This time they were tears of joy. Jamie was going back to school, just as I had silently promised him a year ago. I took the usual home movie of the event, and Jamie's smile filled the lens.

Their going off to school every day drastically affected all of our lives. Jamie's life was the most changed. He loved school. But after a few days in school, it became apparent that his academic performance was more severely limited by his learning disability than by his more obvious physical limitations. Several afternoons a week I went over Jamie's lessons with him a second time at home in order to prepare him for classwork or tests.

I knew his need for this home tutoring would become more intense in each succeeding grade. I no longer clung to false hopes for remaking Jamie. He would always have trouble changing Jello's water. He could learn what he needed for adulthood, but it would require extraordinary effort on his part and on my part. I accepted this new challenge. It would be more attainable than the challenge we had been working so hard at for over a year.

Thus Jamie's studies, even at the second grade level, took priority over brachiating, running and masking. There wasn't enough time in the day to do everything. And if Jamie was going to go to school, he had to do as well as possible. We eliminated the last lingering brachiating, running and masking.

Jamie only went to school now. He did no program. He didn't have any readjustment problem or separation problem. He didn't have any self-image problem either. He was suddenly into Superman, after seeing the latest Christopher Reeve movie, and he wore the red cape I made him and his Superman T-shirt as often as possible. I even caught him wearing the cape under his school clothes a few mornings, with the pair of old black-framed magnifying glasses for his Clark Kent disguise in his pocket. He saw into the refrigerator with his "X-ray vision" and he lifted "boulders" with his powerful hands. I feared, along with millions of other mothers, that my son might think he could really fly off the deck. He planned to use the outfit for his Halloween costume, and even put in an early order for a Superman birthday cake for March.

Jennifer, too, was adjusting to her first time as a full-time student. She had been aware of Jamie's physical problem for a long time, but I suddenly noticed an increase in her sensitivity and compassion for him. One night while I was reading a story to them before turning out the light, Jamie's arm and hand became typically tight and folded up against his chest. I quietly suggested he could just relax and let his hand rest comfortably on his thigh. I put it there and went on reading. A minute or two later his arm had slowly worked its way back up, and he was chewing unconsciously on the cuff of his pajamas. Before I could say anything, Jennifer reached over and gently put Jamie's stiff hand onto her lap and stroked it softly to keep the fingers open.

"To love is to be happy with."

30
Peace

The new treatment might offer nothing which cannot be achieved by other means.

Maslund, 1966, p. 744

The days went by and the Bratts were at peace. There was no more screaming or yelling. There was no more need to justify every decision, action, or opinion to some outside force. Alden handled the rubber and plastics problems of the U.S. Navy and I handled the domestic front. What a pleasure to have happy, sensitive children, free to learn at a comfortable pace, free to sleep later, free to go for a walk, free to play with their family and toys. All that was left to remind us of the program were the holes in the doorway to Jamie's room where the chin-up bar had been, the straight row of shrubs along the old crawl strip, and the ladder bolted to the wall of the playroom—not the therapy room any more. We had returned the patterning table to its owner and had taken down the outdoor ladder. Nobody missed any of it.

We tried to decide if it was a mistake to have gone on the Institutes' program. If we had known about it and not done it, wouldn't we always have wondered if we could have helped Jamie by its methods? We conceded that Jamie did benefit, albeit marginally in comparison to the prospect of total cure. His body was toned up, he had a sport in which he could excel, and he could read and compute with ease. We had taken him off drugs, braces, casts, and abandoned contemplation of unnecessary surgery. But none of these benefits was directly related to the Institutes' techniques. They were obtainable by other methods.

Probably the greatest good that we derived from our involvement with the Institutes was the realization that no one discipline, no one theory, no one person, had all the answers to our problem. And knowing this, we now had the perspective and the will to trust our own judgment about what was best for Jamie.

Probably the greatest harm that we suffered from our involvement with the Institutes was not the lack of results, but the psychological dilemma that we were left with, and that Jamie was left with after constantly being told, either verbally or by implication, that he would be cured or made "better", and then not curing him or making him "better". Every day that we had made him crawl and creep we were in effect saying, "We want to change you, we don't like the way you are." And then when it all failed, and the fantasy of a "better" kid died, everyone had to readjust to the same old kid.

It seemed we had gone from a healthy high as new parents to a healthy low when we had to face Jamie's disability. Then we had abruptly shot up to an unhealthy, unrealistic high when we had read Glenn Doman's book, made three trips to Philadelphia, and dared to hope that Jamie could be cured of cerebral palsy. We had just as abruptly fallen to a correspondingly unhealthy, unrealistic low when we had to admit to ourselves that our son was not going to be cured. From that emotional low point, we could gradually climb back to a realistic, contented position. Alden and I were able to weather these ups and downs. The Institutes was just an experiment that didn't work.

But what about Jamie? Deep down, what did he think of himself and this whole experience? And what did hundreds of other children, whose parents had also given up the program, think of themselves? And what about the brothers and sisters? There were constant rumors among the parents and hints from the Institutes staff of miraculous cures. We had been told outright by several staff members that Jamie could "get well." But we never saw it happen. Not to us, not to any of the families there with us. I wrote to several of the families with whom we had been friendly. Some replied that they too had given up, some replied that they were still plugging along, despite minimal progress to date, and some did not write back.

Did miracles ever really happen there? The Institutes would of course respond defiantly in the affirmative, but I had the feeling that their idea of a miracle was akin to someone taking a perfectly normal baby to the Institutes and if over a period of time the child learned to roll over, then sit up, then to walk, and then to say "Mama," the Institutes would claim credit for each achievement along the way. Even severely brain damaged children could often reach these same goals on their own, though at a delayed pace. We read and were told at the Institutes that the earlier parents put their hurt children on the program the better. Time was the enemy. That is, the Institutes' enemy, we now realized. The younger the child was when beginning the program, the fewer milestones he may already have achieved, and the more were left for the Institutes to claim responsibility for!

Any program short of ignoring a child was bound to help him. Providing a particularly stimulating environment for a normal child or for a brain damaged child was apt to accelerate development to a point. In either case, the child might reach some developmental milestones that he was going to reach anyway sooner. In the case of the brain damaged child, he might be able to reach some milestones that he might not have been able to reach on his own.

But could the extra frequency, intensity, and duration of stimulation bring about performances that were not already within that child's realm of capability? If the child never walked or talked or whatever, then it just wasn't meant to be. What was, was. Not even the Institutes could change that.

Even though Jamie ran well, he still could not willingly wiggle the toes on his right foot. Though he could brachiate well, he could not so much as scratch an itch with his right hand. We had built his body, but there had been no change in his brain cells, no change in function. "Closed brain surgery" (patterning) and the floor program (crawling and creeping) and the cortical organization program (running) had been useless to us. There had been no effect on Jamie's central nervous system.

How then could one determine, particularly in a brain injured child, just what was meant to be? How did we know when we had reached the plateau of an individual's ability or his greatest potential? How hard should we work to find out that potential? Can we ever know? And if we could know that potential, what would be the best program of stimulation to achieve it?

These questions cannot be answered definitively for each child, and that is why desolate parents, who are not ready to accept what their doctors tell them, or what common sense or mother's intuition tell them, keep bringing their hurt children to the Institutes for the Achievement of Human Potential.

Jamie was doing his best for now. With maturity he might make a conscious effort to extend his right arm or to be more organized. But his basic physical disability and learning disability would always be there. There was a limit to his potential, as there was to everyone's. We could accept that now, and work around it. We felt no pressure or regrets about what he couldn't do. It was wiser to put a lift in his shoe and to say things twice to him than to live a stressful life devoted to changing him when changing him was not possible.

Could we have answered these questions about his potential, and reached our new serenity, without following the rigid routine of the program and without experiencing the intense emotional highs and lows that we did?

We thought so. We could have recovered from our initial depression on our own. More easily, in fact, than we recovered from our second depression, the one caused by the program. And Jamie would have progressed on his own at a pace nearly as fast as he did on the program. He would have learned to read by other methods. He would have learned math by other methods. He would have maintained the flexibility and the range of motion of his limbs by other methods. All that crawling, creeping, masking, patterning, and brachiating could only be justified if a child ended up totally cured because of it, or at least significantly changed in a reasonable amount

of time. We neither saw in others nor experienced ourselves such fulfill-
ment. What we saw was a lot of minute progress and a lot of children sitting
up and creeping who would have sat up and crept anyway. Glenn Doman's
spurious remark to our group of parents in the auditorium that, "Here is
where what would have happened anyway happens!" now had a ring of
truth to it.

Even as I thought about all this, I was aware that hundreds of children,
in the United States and around the world, were crawling and creeping
endlessly, and were getting blisters on their hands from the ladder, and that
hundreds of volunteers were filing through people's homes to help with
patterning or whatever new techniques the Institutes was experimenting
with. Parents were forcing their children to endure all this because they
believed what the Institutes staff had told them. They had to believe. No one
would do it otherwise. I had believed, and I had snapped defiantly at
anyone who dared to suggest that we might fail. Then we had worked our
way back to reality and so too would the others in time.

Sometimes I couldn't believe that we had really done it. Or more
accurately, that Jamie had done it. How had he done it? How did he do
anything with only one usable hand? So many times two hands were not
enough for something I was trying to do and I became angry and frustrated.
How angry and frustrated was he inside? Many people complimented me
on my dedication and endurance while conducting the program. But it was
Jamie who endured the demands of the program and who coped so
marvelously with everything in his life. It was Jamie who deserved the
compliments.

I thought that a program of physical and intellectual stimulation for a
hurt child and for a well child was desirable. I thought that Glenn Doman's
program for hurt and well children could accelerate and stimulate the
natural learning process. But a reduced daily requirement, a reevaluation of
the effectiveness of certain techniques, and an honesty about the expected
prognosis were needed. There was too much stress doing the program and
too much stress failing to attain unreasonable requirements. Honesty
would be better. "Your child might walk if we do this", or "Your child might
say three words if we do that", or "Your child will never walk or talk, but
let's see if we can get him to sit up", or "We can slim down your child with
Down Syndrome and teach him some basics, but we can't change his
chromosomes," or "We can teach your child to read at a surprisingly early
age, but its main value will be to impress people, as there is no evidence that
he will maintain that edge over his peers after the first few years in school."

Why didn't they talk like that at the Institutes? Was the staff as deluded
with false hope as were the parents? I was certain there were more failures
than "successes". How many failures did they have to see to be enlightened?
Were they sincere or con artists?

When I reviewed Glenn Doman's book *What to Do About Your Brain-Injured Child*, which was how we originally found out about the Institutes two summers previously, I found that he wrote that, "The objective of such treatment is not to make the child a happy or successful cripple, but instead to make him a non-cripple, in both physical and intellectual terms... The majority of brain injured children we are seeing today are markedly and measurably improved". (p. 243) In his lectures he even talked about actually hastening evolution by making well kids "weller" with his methods. These are broad goals and bold assertions. On other pages he was more realistic. "The results, therefore, will range from total success to total failure". (p. 3) And Glenn Doman even portrayed himself as deeply caring. "Ever intruding on my thoughts are the kids who fail, even today, and they are far too many, and there remain a few who are actually not changed at all". (p. 266)

I felt he had his quantifiers, "the majority" and "a few", reversed. And I doubted that Jamie ever intruded on his thoughts.

Glenn Doman would probably defend his application of the theory of neurological organization by accusing us of not doing the program long enough. Ten years was not long enough in at least one case that we knew about.

Or he might use another weak defense: to get some "delinquent" parents to do anything at all for their hurt children, they had to be lied to; or at the other end of the spectrum, that the program gave some devoted parents a sense of doing something for their hurt children. However, most other parents of hurt children, ourselves included, would rather pursue varied interests, of value to them as well as to the child, rather than to steadily deplete their monetary resources and their stamina trying to reach an unattainable goal.

Glenn Doman might point to his research and his "success" stories to defend his theories. I would point out that if my child had been cured by the Institutes' program I would have told them to give my name and address and phone number to anyone who came to them, and I would have vouched for the validity of the program. I would have shouted it to the world. I would have hired a sky writer. But they flatly refused to give us any such names when we asked. We heard no shouting. We saw no sky writing.

I was leaning on the cedar post fence between the two spruce trees in our front yard. Benjiman, already one and a half years old, was sitting in the car with Daddy, who had just returned from his regular Saturday golf match. Benjiman was going "Vroom, vroom" and pretending to drive, just as Jamie had done at that age. But Daddy wasn't paying much attention to Benjiman at the moment. He was instead watching in awe the spectacle on the road in front of our house.

Jennifer, now almost six, was riding her bicycle back and forth by the car, making skillful U-turns. She was riding beautifully, having easily mastered in a few afternoons the balance and rhythm required to make the transition from training wheels to two wheels.

Jamie too was proudly riding his bicycle alongside her all by himself— and without training wheels!

Jennifer desperately wanted her big brother to be able to do what she could do. In the two weeks since she had been able to ride alone, she had helped Jamie every day on his bike, from which we had removed the training wheels at their insistence. I had heard her praise him lavishly as he dared to coast from a little higher up on our downhill driveway each time.

"Good, Jamie, good. You didn't even tip over that time. Now try it from that tree."

"Great, Jamie! Now try to keep both feet on the pedals as long as possible. Go up to the rock garden this time." Jamie obeyed her every command and concentrated on this task harder then he ever concentrated on brachiating.

This morning, they both got up early and went outside to practice. At 9:00 Jennifer called me out to see what Jamie could do. He was pedaling a few feet at the bottom of the driveway before crashing into the garage door! I got out the movie camera and he performed this feat over and over for me.

We decided he was ready to try the flat road. After several tries, he managed to go many shaky yards before having to put his feet down on the pavement. Then he would start up again and go a little further. His right foot was awkward on its pedal, as if he had on a ski boot. He occasionally tipped over because he couldn't protect himself by throwing out his right foot if he had leaned too far to the right, and he couldn't shift his weight to the right to counteract an unexpected tip to the left. But his right hand stayed marvelously in place on the handlebar grip. By midafternoon he was riding almost 200 yards without stopping. A confirmed rider, I was tempted to say. He had been anxious for Daddy to return home so he could show him what he could do. For Jamie it was his greatest accomplishment ever, because it did for him what a million brachiates could never do. It made him a regular guy.

I was leaning on the fence thinking about all this, and more, when Jamie rode triumphantly by at top speed, and yelled, "Look Ma, two hands!"

Afterword

May 1986

Several years have past since the events I wrote of took place. As I write this, it is spring 1986 and Jamie is 12 years old and finishing sixth grade. He receives average grades in a regular classroom, plays trumpet in the school band, collects Masters of the Universe toys, has attained purple belt level of competence in karate, and, like every school child, is looking forward to summer vacation. Jennifer is 10 ½ years old and finishing fifth grade. She reads voraciously, is extremely artistically inclined like my sister, and is taking guitar and clarinet lessons. Benjiman is six years old and is finishing kindergarten. He is a "Toys R Us Kid" and has lost his first tooth. He doesn't remember the program at all.

I am into my fourth year back at teaching, and am finishing a two year course of study at the University of New Hampshire leading to a Master's Degree in Early Childhood Special Needs. Alden has done most of the housework, meal preparation, and child care for these two years while I studied. He says that being on the patterning program was good training for this role, as he did similar chores while I kept Jamie crawling and creeping back then.

As part of my graduate program, I investigated the professional and popular literature concerning the Institutes for the Achievement of Human Potential, its theory of neurological organization, and Glenn Doman, the founder and force behind the Institutes. As a parent desperately searching for help for my son in 1979, it never occurred to me then to look for any professional evaluation of patterning. I read Doman's book, and wanted to believe it. I was blind because of my hope and my love. I didn't know critical journal articles existed. I suspect that most parents of impaired children are not aware of, or at least have not personally read, the substantial amount of professional literature that does in fact exist about the Institutes. A review of that body of literature, as well as of the supportive books and articles written by Institutes staff and friends, is the purpose of the appendix which follows.

This research has resolved many lingering questions for Alden and myself. We let go of the program slowly in 1981, not wanting to make a mistake or to appear foolish. For many months, whenever we were asked about the success of the program, we listed off Jamie's gains, as if the Institutes were responsible. Whenever parents who had heard about us called us to ask if they should take their child to Philadelphia, (there were several), I was honest in saying that Jamie was not cured. But I did not discourage them from following in our footsteps. I did not want to snatch away their hope and I did not want them to think that I was bitter. And I was undecided about the true intentions and credibility of the Institutes' staff.

Time, and writers such as Melvyn P. Robbins, Roger D. Freeman, Edward Zigler, and Robin Warshaw, have changed all that. I know where I stand philosophically and emotionally. I do not feel guilt or failure for having quit the program. Rather I feel embarrassment and anger for ever having gone on the program at all. My only guilt is for forcing Jamie to endure the indignity and the pain. I would now do all I could to prevent other families from making our mistake. I would tell them our story and I would quote the research and I would write in the sky: Don't do it!

I quoted Glenn Doman as saying to us that the reason parents accept the program more readily than do professionals is that parents have "less to unlearn." He is essentially gloating over parents' lack of information and their susceptibility to his program, without making it sound derogatory. After all, without susceptible parents there would be no Institutes for the Achievement of Human Potential.

Parents must be informed. Studies that attempt to replicate IAHP methods invite criticism from the Institutes. Rather, more brutally honest personal stories of families who have actually followed the regimen as prescribed by the Institutes need to be revealed. Their stories can have the greatest impact. Doman has written. Professionals have written. Now is the time for families who have been on the program to write.

Appendix

A Review of the Literature on the Institutes for the Achievement of Human Potential

May 1986

> *We must insist upon ferreting out fact from fiction.*
> Robbins & Glass, 1969, p. 323

This review will be in five parts, and will consider both the positive and negative evaluations of the Institutes. I will first review the books and journal articles written by Glenn Doman and other staff members or supporters of the Institutes for the Achievement of Human Potential (IAHP), all of which promote the theory and methods of the program. Then I will review the books written by parents who have used the patterning program with their own disabled children, which are also positive in their ultimate evaluation of patterning. The third section of this review will be on other articles appearing in newspapers and magazines in support of parents implementing the program.

Finally, I will review the critical evaluations of the Institutes, which include professional journal articles written by other than Institutes staff members, and one magazine article. The purpose of the scientific literature, in contrast to some of the more subjective literature reviewed first, is:

> ...to apply standards of evidence to the assumptions which underlie the theory of neurological organization and to experimental data cited in support of the purported relationship between reading and neurological organization. The analysis is an attempt to reach a rational conclusion concerning the merits of the theory. ...The scientific and professional community have standards which remain unaffected by the publicity surrounding a theory. If the theory of neurological organization is to be taken seriously by the scholarly community, then its advocates are under an obligation to provide reasonable support for the tenets of the theory and a series of experimental investigations, consistent with current scientific standards, which test the efficacy of the rationale (Robbins & Glass, 1969, p. 369).

Most parents and parent supporters unfortunately do not encounter these latter writings.

Favorable Books and Reviews

Institutes-Sponsored Publications

My first introduction to the Institutes was Glenn Doman's book, *What to Do About Your Brain-Injured Child*. Actually, the full title of the book, which takes up the entire cover, is *What to Do About Your Brain-Injured Child or Your Brain Damaged, Mentally Retarded, Mentally Deficient, Cerebral Palsied, Spastic, Flaccid, Rigid, Epileptic, Autistic, Athethoid, Hyperactive Child*. It is skillfully, logically, and convincingly written. That is what got us to Philadelphia, where we found the author's spoken words to be even more mesmerizing than his written words. But that book, published in 1974, was not the first book dealing with the Institutes' theory and methods. There were at least a dozen previously published.

Carl Delacato, an educator who first used the term "neurological organization" and who was Doman's early partner from 1947 to the 1960s, wrote *The Treatment and Prevention of Reading Problems, The Neuropsychological Approach* in 1959, *The Diagnosis and Treatment of Speech and Reading Problems* in 1963, and *Neurological Organization and Reading* in 1966. In the second book he explained how creeping and the use of a trampoline recreates the stages of neurological development. A review of the book in *Neurology* said, "It is of passing interest if viewed as an excursion into the realm of science fiction" (quoted in Bird, 1967, p. 74). In the third book, Delacato wrote about "flip-flops," or patterning, as a treatment procedure.

The theory of neurological organization states that superior cortical development, measured by mobility and intelligence, is reached only by the individual organism's nervous system mimicking each of the phylogenetic or evolutionary stages of development, from medulla to pons to midbrain to initial cortex to early cortex to primitive cortex to sophisticated cortex, or from fish to amphibian to reptile to primate to man. If an organism skips any stage for whatever reason, he will be incapable of perfectly performing the abilities associated with that skipped stage and all subsequent stages. These abilities are outlined in the Institutes' Developmental Profile and Chart of Human Neurological Organization.

A child who has skipped or improperly completed a stage will need to be forcibly brought back to that stage by the techniques described earlier in Part II of this book. Imposing the evolutionary patterns of movement—crawling, creeping, brachiating, and patterning, along with other treatment procedures designed to increase the brain's receptivity to all this—on a brain injured or neurologically disorganized child results in normal brain organization and corresponding skills.

In 1967, John R. Kerschner wrote *An Investigation of the Doman-Delacato Theory of Neuropsychology as It Applies to Training Mentally Retarded Children in Public Schools*. It projects a somewhat positive view of the program, and because of that was sharply criticized by R. D. Freeman, a vehement member of the opposition. In *The Journal of Pediatrics*, Freeman (1967) said that experimental bias affected both teachers and parents in the study. Since they had all heard in the popular press that improvements were possible, they expected and therefore saw progress in the experimental group, but did not have the same enthusiasm for the control group, and therefore saw no progress.

James M. Wolf, Ed.D., wrote *Temple Fay, Progenitor of the Doman-Delacato Procedures* in 1968. Temple Fay was a neurosurgeon who was Doman's mentor and idol. Fay's work laid the groudwork for liquid balance and masking, two treatment procedures used by the Institutes.

In 1968, Evan Thomas, who was then Medical Director of the Children's Evaluation Institute of the Institutes for the Achievement of Human Potential, published *Brain-Injured Children, with Special Reference to Doman-Delacato Methods of Treatment*. It is a description of the theory, the Profile, and the five treatment principles of the Institutes.

Edwin B. LeWinn, then Director of the Institutes for Clinical Investigation, wrote *Human Neurological Organization* in 1969. This book is an in-depth explanation and justification of the theory that is the foundation of Glenn Doman's program. He related the history of the Institutes, and cited studies of the effect of increased environmental stimulation on performance and on brain structure. LeWinn believes, as does Glenn Doman, that such stimulation "grows the brain."

Glenn Doman has written more books than just the 1974 what-to-do book. He published *How to Teach Your Baby to Read* in 1964, which explained the flashcard system, and *How to Teach Your Baby Math* in 1974, which explains the dot program. *How to Multiply Your Baby's Intelligence*, which appeared in 1984, on which Doman was working when we were on the program, explains his rationale for the frequency and intensity of early stimulation of all children. *How to Give Your Baby Encyclopedic Knowledge* was published in 1985 and is co-authored with his daughter Janet Doman (now the Director of the IAHP; her father is Chairman of the Board) and Susan Aisen. This work gives specific instructions for making bits of intelligence cards and programs of intelligence cards. Doman, according to the latter publication, is now working on a multivolume encyclopedia of sensory stimulation. He has also authored or overseen the preparation of numerous booklets on all aspects of the IAHP for distribution to parents on the program, including a monthly magazine called *In Report*, which contains feature articles and progress notes on children currently on the program.

In addition to these books, there are two papers that were published by Institutes staff members, one in a professional journal and one in an educational textbook. "Children with Severe Injuries, Neurological Organization in Terms of Mobility." by Robert J. Doman, M.D., Eugene B. Spitz, M.D., Elizabeth Zucman, M.D., Carl Delacato, Ed.D., and Glenn Doman, P.T., appeared in the *Journal of the American Medical Association* (1960). The study reported in this paper extends Delacato's (1959) hypothesis of the relationship between neurological organization and reading to the relationship of neurological organization to mobility. The treatment group consisted of 76 brain-injured children ranging in chronological age from 12 months to nine years, and the treatment program consisted of various amounts of daily creeping, crawling and patterning. All children showed improvement in mobility after six to 20 months of treatment. The authors reported that 56 of the original 76 had been nonwalkers at the outset, and that 11 of those walked at the end of this program. The encouraging results of this study, in the authors' eyes, combined with their understanding that brain injury is in the brain and not in the distant, uninjured limbs, led to the formalization of the Institutes' theory of human neurological organization (Delacato's 1966 book and LeWinn's 1969 book), and to the invention of an instrument to assess brain-injured children—The Developmental Profile.

The other paper, "Neurological Organization: The Basis for Learning" by Edwin B. LeWinn, M.D., Glenn Doman, Sc.D., Robert J. Doman, M.D., Carl Delacato, Ed.D., Eugene Spitz, M.D., and Evan W. Thomas, M.D., was published as a chapter in Jerome Hellmuth's book *Learning Disorders* (1966). It explains brain growth, brain stimulation, brain potential, brain injury, and the five treatment principles and 22 treatment procedures then used at the IAHP.

One more book by a staff member is not specifically about the IAHP, but it is related. Raymond Dart, an African anthropologist, wrote *Adventures with the Missing Link* in 1959. It concerns his discovery of a human ancestor located evolutionarily between the creeping apes and the upright apes: the swinging or brachiating ape. After Doman met Dart during one of his expeditions to study primitive societies in Africa, he invited Dart to join his staff in Philadelphia in 1966, heading The Institute of Man, created specifically for Dart. Once Doman figured out a way—via the overhead ladder—to reproduce that newly discovered evolutionary stage in man's development, all children on the program were thenceforth given the opportunity for adventures with the missing link. Dart's *Adventures with the Missing Link* was republished by The Institutes Press in 1967, with an introduction by Glenn Doman.

Dart's work, like Doman's, met with some initial skepticism. Doman's consoling introductory remarks could easily be interpreted as Doman's hope for future validation of his own work:

> But Dart's discovery—and the conclusion he drew from it— met no easy acceptance. It challenged the preconceptions of most of the then highest eminences of the scientific establishment. With but few exceptions, they turned upon him with uninformed skepticism, disputed the facts and challenged his conclusions. Like Kepler, Columbus, Galileo, and Darwin, he had to endure the scorn of fossilized minds who, having once refused to recognize a fact, than felt compelled to hold to the curious consistency of rejecting a hundred, a thousand, and ultimately, an avalanche of facts. Be it said to their credit, however, at least some of these men, after two decades or more of fevered opposition, finally mustered the courage and the much-delayed grace to acknowledge publicly their errors, as others before them had grudgingly conceded that the world was not flat or that the sun and stars did not revolve around our little planet embedded in transparent, glassy spheres (p. xv-xvi).

In a recent personal communication with an anthropologist, I have learned that while Dart's discovery of Australopithecine man is indeed considered a significant contribution to the field, his particular characterization of the habits of Australopithecines and where he places them on the evolutionary time line remains controversial today.

Books by Parents

Interspersed amongst the history of these textbooks and journal articles about the IAHP are personal accounts. Five parents have written favorably about the Institutes. Peggy Napear described her daughter Janey's 12 trips to Philadelphia from October 1965 to April 1972 in *Brain Child, A Mother's Diary* (1974). Janey's program was nowhere near as strenuous as ours, and Napear even revealed that they did not so some parts as directed. At the end, Janey did not talk distinctly, and was just beginning to walk—yet a staff member predicted that she would be ready for ballet in a year.

Elizabeth Peiper wrote *Sticks and Stones, The Story of a Loving Child* (undated) about her son with mental retardation. The book is only partly about the Institutes, and is mostly about her feelings as a mother of a disabled child, and her decision to institutionalize her child. It is not particularly favorable to the Institutes, but neither is it critical.

William Breisky extolled the virtues of the program in his 1974 tale of his daughter Karen's success, but not cure, in *I Think I Can*. It is a moving story of an unexpected tragedy and the ensuing search for help, and of parental dedication. It ends with Doman's dramatic presentation of her case history to the Sixteenth Constitutional Convention of the United Steelworkers of America in 1972. That organization has been a substantial financial supporter of the IAHP since 1968, the same year a negative statement by the American Academy for Cerebral Palsy, and several other medical associations (see the section of this chapter headed Criticisms) ended foundation funds for the Institutes. The Steelworkers' only requirement for their continued generosity is that Doman present a success story each year at their convention.

A review of books about the IAHP would not be complete without mentioning the work of David Melton, who has been almost as prolific and powerful with his pen as has been Glenn Doman. He wrote *Todd* in 1968, about his brain injured son and their experiences with the program. The book seems to be more of a propaganda tool for the Institutes than a personal story as it is mostly an exact reiteration of Doman's lectures. Todd's status and future prognosis is unclear at the conclusion, but Melton's opinions and convictions concerning the Institutes are crystal clear. This is the book that I bought several copies of and distributed among my patterners as explanation and justification of our need for their services. I thought then that it was a wonderfully concise and moving story. I wrote a letter to Melton inquiring as to Todd's adult status. I got no reply.

Further evidence of Melton's devotion to the Institutes is the fact that the introduction to *Todd* was written by Glenn Doman, and, reciprocally, when Doman published his how-to book in 1974, Melton, a commercial artist, provided the illustrations. Melton wrote three more books about the Institutes, and collaborated on a fourth. In 1972 *A Child Called Hopeless* was published, which is a fictional account of a family that decides to go on the program and the sacrifices they must make—through the eyes of a seventh grade sister. It was written specifically for siblings of families engaged in the program, again reiterating Doman's philosophy. In 1976 Melton published *How to Help Your Preschooler Learn More...Faster...and Better*. This too is Glenn Doman's ideas and words, this time concerning well children and their insatiable need for early knowledge about everything. According to Melton, the ideal way for children to be taught is by mothers at home. In Chapter 10 he writes, "Should you send your preschooler to preschool or a daycare center? Only if the other choices are leaving him in a lion's cage, a shark-infested surf, or a burning building" (p. 181).

David Melton worked with Raymundo Veras to produce *Children of Dreams, Children of Hope* in 1975. Veras was a physician in Brazil whose son, paralyzed from a diving accident, regained considerable movement after being on the Institutes' program. Veras was so grateful and convinced of the program's validity that he wrote a book and opened a rehabilitation clinic in Brazil using Doman's methods. And Doman regularly confers on staff members "The Brazilian Medal of Honor," which has no endorsement from the government of Brazil (Warshaw, 1982, p. 185).

In Part II of his book, Veras went a step further than simple admiration and restatement of Doman's work. Chapter 21 is entitled: "How to Make Mongoloids Well." This is an unfortunate use of an outdated term. Down Syndrome has been the accepted term for more than ten years, especially in the field of mental retardation. Children with Down Syndrome were in our class, but they were always referred to as Veras Babies. Veras proposed in that chapter that "mongoloids" are not brain-deficient but rather that the abnormal chromosome count is caused by tension, smoking, and poor nutrition, such as the consumption of coke, hamburgers, and coffee, during pregnancy. He claimed that patterning can make these children well. He claimed that some of them could go to universities, should get married, and might have genius potential. "The goal for our mongoloids is normality and nothing less" (p. 199). Such statements sell books.

Newspaper and Magazine Articles

The popular press has produced much publicity for Doman's work with both brain injured children and well children (The Better Baby Institute). For example, a newspaper in the town next to mine, *The York Weekly*, ran a front page story with pictures, on March 12, 1984, by Helen Pettay, headlined "Therapy Plan Turns into One Family's Adventure." I met and visited with the family a few weeks after that. I was at that time guardedly honest about my experience, and did not judge or advise. A bigger, more prestigious newspaper, *The New York Times*, printed pictures and a story by Barbara Campbell on page one, on April 16, 1976, entitled, "60 Volunteers a Week Aid Retarded Boy."

I telephoned this family one evening. Ten years later and with a still uncured son, the mother had only words of praise for the Institutes. She said, "It's a drag having a brain injured child, but it's not fair to direct one's anger at the Institutes. ...The Institutes gave me a wonderful feeling of control instead of helplessness." She reported that one of her volunteers went on to become a senior staff member at the Institutes. She herself now had three graduate degrees in education. Her son is no longer on the program, and she described him as having "increased spatial awareness, able to compute with ease, able to read large print, and tuned in to people," all qualities that she did not see in the children she taught as a former special education teacher. One of her most descriptive statements was her comment that her home had been furnished in "early neurological."

"Miracle in Pennsylvania," by Paul Ernst, appeared in the September 1962 issue of *Good Housekeeping*. It told of the slow but seemingly miraculous improvement of David Posnett, who was hit by a car, and then entered into the program. "In three [years] he should be a normal, active boy again" it predicted (p. 38). The Institutes received a great deal of positive publicity from this one case. Several other articles on the family were written. The Institutes made a movie of the Posnett home and programming, and regularly showed it to parents during the initial evaluation week. We watched it in April 1980. Warshaw (1982) reveals that this hope of normalcy was never realized.

Joan Beck wrote a two-part piece for *The Chicago Tribune Sunday Magazine*, September 13 and 27, 1964, entitled "Mental Miracles for Brain-Injured Children" and "Why Johnny Can Read," respectively. Beck introduced the first article with, "Scientists in Philadelphia are not only saving hundreds of mentally crippled children from lives of blackout and isolation but are actually teaching many of them to outperform their normal brothers and sisters" (p. 26). One of the case histories that she mentioned was of the late Ambassador Joseph P. Kennedy. He was still unable to walk and talk 2 ½ years after a stroke and treatment with traditional symptomatic methods, but after one month at the IAHP he left walking and talking, Beck reported (p. 29). I wrote to Senator Edward Kennedy asking if this was true. He did not write back. The rest of the article gives an accurate history of the development of the Institutes and the treatment principles. It includes many direct Doman quotes. "We define wellness the same way you do—a normal child. Anything less than that we consider a failure" (p. 38). He went on to say that one of the reasons for failure is that parents may not do the program as described. Beck's second piece, subtitled "Great Challenges to Modern Medicine," asserts that reading problems can best be prevented and treated not by traditional speech therapy or remedial reading but rather by the neurological approach—that is, by a huge dose of creeping.

John Bird's 1967 article in *The Saturday Evening Post*, "When Children Can't Learn," again gives the usual background on brain growth, stages of neurological organization, and a successful case history. "Some medics and teachers see the concept of neurological organization as a possible breakthrough... . Dozens of schools have established special classes in which children with learning problems crawl, creep and practice visual exercises for certain periods of the day" (pp. 28, 30). There is an amazing full page picture of a large class of children creeping in a school gym in New York City.

"Hope for Brain-Injured Children," by Albert Q. Maisel, appeared in the October 1964 issue of *Reader's Digest*. It is similar to many of the articles I have just reviewed, giving the history of the IAHP and a case study.

There are many more magazine articles and news stories similar to those I have mentioned. Lately, though, the emphasis in the press has been on The Better Baby Institute, which is Doman's effort to make normal children into "geniuses." Joni Winn, in "Boosting Baby's IQ," in *The Saturday Evening Post,* November 1983, wrote that "Doman's robust enthusiasm endears him to eager-eyed parents who follow him as a modern Pied Piper" (p. 104). Lynn Langway, in "Bringing up Superbaby," the cover story in Newsweek, March 28, 1983, acknowledged that learning pressure on tiny tots may shortchange emotional and cognitive growth, and concluded that we had better not exclude "babbling and bouncing" in infancy.

Criticisms

Scientific Literature

Melvyn P. Robbins, Ph.D., is a confirmed critic of patterning. In April 1966, "A Study of the Validity of Delacato's Theory of Neurological Organization" appeared in *Exceptional Children,* following the publication of Delacato's three books on the subject. This article reports the findings of a study in which Robbins attempted to prove or disprove the relationship between functional ability and anatomical development, or, more specifically, to answer the question whether ability or inability in reading and speech are directly related to creeping and laterality. Delacato's treatment was added to a normal second grade class, with two control groups, one receiving no treatment and one receiving a different treatment. The experimenters were trained in methods at the IAHP. The results revealed no more differences in reading between the groups than would be expected by chance. Reading was not enhanced by the program. And Robbins concluded, "Since the central concept of the theory—the relationship between neurological organization and reading—has not been supported by the findings, the entire theory is suspect" (p. 523).

Delacato responded to this article in a letter in the November 1966 *Exceptional Children.* He pointed out what he considered to be defects in Robbins's study, with special emphasis on the random selection of treatment as opposed to an individually designed program, and the lack of intensity of programming. In the same issue, in a letter of reply to Delacato, Robbins refuted Delacato's objections, criticized Delacato's studies, and then offered, "I suggest Mr. Delacato join with me in a major research project.... I am eagerly awaiting Mr. Delacato's response to this proposal" (p. 200). No subsequent project was undertaken.

Robbins also studied retarded readers. "Test of the Doman-Delacato Rationale with Retarded Readers" was published in *JAMA,* October 3, 1967. His conclusion was that creeping was only good for poor creepers.

In 1969, Robbins and Gene V. Glass, Ph.D., reviewed the results of the two earlier Robbins studies and responded to the earlier paper by Institutes staff members (LeWinn, Doman, Doman, Delacato, Spitz, & Thomas, 1966) in a previous Hellmuth book. In a new Hellmuth book Robbins and Glass wrote a chapter entitled "The Doman-Delacato Rationale: A Critical Analysis." They explained the theory in detail and then criticized several of its foundations. Specifically, they indicated that the idea that ontogeny could recapitulate phylogeny had long been discredited in education and psychology. Individual members of a species in fact grow more and more dissimilar from their ancestors over time, especially after the fetal stage. Doman and Delacato, though, extend the theory into childhood and adulthood. They argued the human infant never shows any ability to climb nor is he ever a pure quadruped, as were our phylogenetic ancestors. They also disputed sequential development, brain stages, and localization of functions. Humans have been known to skip stages with no ill effects and to function normally after surgical removal of large portions of the brain. The necessity for unilateral cerebral dominance was questioned too, because mixed laterality occurs frequently in the normal population. Robbins and Glass cited recent studies that indicate that stuttering and other speech and reading problems are not due to lack of dominance. At the end of the paper, Robbins and Glass evaluated 11 positive studies on the relationship between neurological organization and reading. All 11 "are exemplary for their faults...were naively designed and clumsily analyzed...and executed and reported in an atmosphere of relative insensitivity to basic considerations of empirical, experimental research" (p. 347).

Richard Masland, M.D., then Director of the National Institutes of Neurological Diseases and Blindness, wrote "Unproven Methods of Treatment" in *Pediatrics* in May 1966. He didn't mention IAHP, but he was clearly referring to that program because he wrote of crawling, creeping and neurological organization. He acknowledged two shortcomings of the average physician: preoccupation with diagnosis so that parents turn elsewhere for assistance, and a tendency to offer too early and too dogmatic a prognosis and therapy, unintentionally limiting therapeutic efforts. Masland stated that:

> We in the profession have two serious and continuing responsibilties. The first is to assure that every neurologically deviant child, however deficient he may appear, receive not only a full diagnosis and therapeutic workup, but also a supervised and continuing program of remediation....The second is to develop a program whereby existing and proposed methods of remediation can be subjected to critical scientific evaluation (p. 714).

Roger D. Freeman, M.D., published "Controversy Over 'Patterning' as a Treatment for Brain Damage in Children" in *JAMA*, October 30, 1967. He listed nine controversies associated with the Institutes' methods. They are:

1. The Institutes overlooks the natural, or clinical, course of development of some brain injured children. Glenn Doman said in his lectures to us that before his treatment methods were developed he had never heard of a single brain injured child getting well. In fact, he said and has written that children left on the floor to creep and crawl do better than children receiving conventional treatment. Yet many experienced physicians, wrote Freeman, have been witness to spontaneous and unexplained partial and complete recoveries in children severely delayed and not receiving treatment of any kind. Such recoveries might randomly occur in children on the program, with the improvement mistakenly attributed to patterning.
2. The Institutes asserts its methods treat the brain, but there is no scientific proof that patterning has any effect whatsoever on the central nervous system.
3. The Institutes states that brain potential is unknown and that even a defective child may have above average ability. Desperate parents cling to this hope, and if improvement is seen, which may only be due to the child's clinical course, it is credited to the Institues' regimen.
4. The Institutes requires parents to become therapists, which may jeopardize the parent-child relationship and place the burden of failure on parents.
5. The Institutes actively prevents young children who have not mastered crawling and creeping from engaging in such age-appropriate activities as standing, walking, sitting, or rolling by the use of specific devices strapped onto their bodies. The value and long and short term effects of this procedure are unproven.
6. The Institutes makes statements which arouse parental anxiety. For example, there is a constant warning in publications and lectures that children not receiving the Institutes' programming are likely to die earlier. Glenn Doman's first lecture to us told of a family who finally had come to the Institues, and the child, so close to treatment, died in a hotel room. The tone in which parents are bluntly told that common child-rearing practices, such as snug clothing, blank walls, or confinement to playpens, are damaging, is overly alarming. Furthermore, the rigidity required in the performance of all parts of the program leads parents to fear they might be impeding their child's progress if they deviate in the least.
7. The Institutes assumes any improvements that occur in a child are due to the specific program elements. Yet there are so many uncontrollable variables, from rekindled hope to increased sensory stimulation where none may have existed before, to community support and involvement,

that can account for the child's improved performance.

8. The assessment instrument used by the Institutes is neither as simple, conclusive, or as valid as it is claimed to be.

9. There are indefensible statistical defects in studies done by Institues staff.

Freeman concluded:

> Since a well-controlled study which would study all aspects of the controversy regarding effectiveness of the program of the Institutes is probably impossible to design and carry out at this time, physicians and other professionals will have to weigh carefully the recommendation of such treatment (p. 388).

In May 1968, the *Journal of Pediatrics* published a joint official statement from the American Academy for Cerebral Palsy, the Canadian Association for Children with Learning Disabilities, the Canadian Association for Retarded Children, the Canadian Rehabilitation Council for the Disabled, the American Congress of Rehabilitation Medicine, the National Association for Retarded Children, and the American Academy of Physical Medicine and Rehabilitation, which had been previously published in other journals as well. The statement summarizes the theory and studies done as of that date, and lists concerns similar to those noted by Freeman. They added a concern about the promotional methods used by the Institutes which make it nearly impossible for parents to refuse treatment without calling into question their adequacy as parents. The statement mentions that a properly designed, comprehensive study was in the final stages of planning when the Institutes backed out of the agreement to participate. With this action the burden of proof lay with the Institutes.

Herbert S. Cohen, M.D., Herbert G. Birch, M.D., and Lawrence T. Taft, M.D., published "Some Considerations for Evaluating the Doman-Delacato 'Patterning' Method" in *Pediatrics*, February 1970. They remarked that any method that claimed to make normal children out of disabled children and to make geniuses out of normal children "must be subjected to the most careful scrutiny" (p. 302). They cautioned that in so doing:

> One must not be provoked by innacuracies and extravagances which, sometimes in the heat of controversy and as a result of zeal, may have been made by both the advocates and adversaries of the method. In our effort to evaluate the worth of the patterning method, we shall try to insulate ourselves from emotional reactions that may be stimulated by verbal exchanges. Our emphasis will be upon the facts (p. 303).

Any therapeutic method, they asserted, must be assessed on two levels, the theoretical and the empirical. "The history of biology is replete with considerations of the weaknesses of recapitulationist theory" (p. 304), but "A failure to find support for a treatment method in basic science does not in itself justify the rejection of a practice" (pp. 304-305). Therefore, one must consider the value of patterning from an empirical viewpoint only. Since the method was new, the authors felt that its evaluation had to derive from the data published by the Institutes' 1960 study as reported in *JAMA*. Although improvement in mobility was reported for all 76 subjects, of the 56 nonambulatory children, 45 were still not walking at the end of treatment, and of the 11 who did achieve ambulation, nine were under the age of two at the onset of treatment. "Clearly, maturational factors independent of the treatment regimen could have resulted in similar changes, especially in the very young patients" (p. 306). The authors cited findings from their own clinic of children achieving independent walking after having received no special therapeutic programs, though with significant delay. Given this,

> The results reported by the advocates of patterning appear to be singularly unimpressive and lead to the possible inference that the reported changes were at least as much a function of maturation over time as they were improvement induced by treatment (p. 306).

The authors also compared their own clinic results with data from one of Delacato's studies of the effect of patterning on speech development. Again they found the percentile improvement figure was nearly identical for both groups. The authors comment:

> The comparative figures on locomotion development and on speech progress should not be taken literally. The cases in our clinic and those to whom patterning was applied may of course have been different from one another. They are presented less in a spirit of refutation than as an illustration of the need to have comparable data on an appropriately selected control group, if the changes attributed to therapy in children exhibiting delays in development are to be meaningfully assessed (p. 307).

Cohen, Birch, and Taft discussed several other problems which would discount the positive effects of patterning on increases in IQ scores in preschoolers, again mentioning the positive impacts of an improved environment and increased stimulation provided by almost any treatment. Their conclusion was that more scientific studies are needed

> ...before 'patterning' or any other method may claim sufficient

universal applicability to serve as the sole therapeutic approach to one or more disturbances in intellectual and motor functioning (p. 313).

Ronald Neman et al. (1975), a research team based at the National Association for Retarded Children (ARC/N) applied patterning to 66 institutionalized mentally retarded children and reported some minor gains, but "No dramatic cases of individual improvement were observed" (p. 381). This statement outraged Edward Zigler and Victoria Seitz. Two months later, in the same journal, *American Journal of Mental Deficiency* (March 1975), they replied. The tone of their response was incredulity that the "no findings" report did not more resoundingly discredit patterning. Zigler and Seitz feared that some parents might misinterpret ARC/N's position as support for patterning. The authors criticized specific aspects of the study, such as subject selection and the statistical analysis, and stated that:

Any human treatment should be first assessed against the principle of Primum non nocere (First not to injure).... This principle must be expanded not only to a concern about whether a treatment injures the individuals to whom it is applied, but also the effects on the families of the recipients of the treatment (p. 490).

Neman replied in the same issue, stating that Zigler's preconceived bias against patterning influenced his critique. Neman took Zigler's complaints and refuted them or defended himself.

Since Neman's study was with mildly and moderately retarded children only, Zigler and Sara Sparrow subsequently studied patterning's effects with severely and profoundly retarded institutionalized children. They published their results, "Evolution of a Patterning Treatment for Retarded Children," in *Pediatrics*, August 1978. This study was conducted with three groups of 15 children each, four females and 11 males, totaling 45 subjects. The experimenters were trained at the Institutes, whose staff Zigler and Sparrow described as "most cooperative." The treatment group received a program of masking, brachiating, patterning, crawling and creeping for one year. A matched group did success-oriented motivational activities with foster grandparents, such as using music and manipulative toys. The third group received no treatment. On a wide range of behavioral measures, the majority of the 45 children showed no gains from pretest to posttest. In conclusion, the authors stated that "The patterning treatment investigated in this study cannot be recommended for severely retarded children" (p. 137).

Zigler, like Robbins a dozen years before him, did not remain silent. In

July 1981, his paper "A Plea to End the use of the Patterning Treatment for Retarded Children" was published in the *American Journal of Orthopsychiatry*. It is concise and thorough, and especially appropriate for parents, educators, and therapists who may not want to get into statistical and theoretical issues. Zigler berated the popular press for its failure to "even allude to the fact that a controvery over the value of patterning has raged in the scientific journals for twenty years" (p. 388), and he shamed the professionals who "must take some of the blame for offering so little hope and emotional support that parents would turn to a treatment of such questionable worth" (p. 388). He was concerned that there is still no independent scientific data on patterning and he was bewildered at the lay person's lack of suspicion. He resented the popular press focus on families just beginning the program, full of enthusiasm and hope. He wrote, "I know of no accounts relating the experiences of families some time after they have assayed or completed the treatment" (p. 389). Referring to the treatment by foster grandparents in his study, he believed that "Maturation and basic human interaction may account for many of the gains often attributed to patterning" (p. 389). Zigler offered ideas for alternative treatments, such as behavior modification and early intervention. He ended by stating, "We do not counsel abandoning hope, but neither do we suggest grasping at straws. The old saw about the cure being worse than the disease may prove sadly true for the families who try patterning" (p. 390). Dr. Zigler and Dr. Robert N. Hodapp are about to publish *Understanding Mental Retardation*, which will iterate this appraisal of patterning.

W. Herbert published a short piece entitled "Treatment for Brain Damage Under Fire" in *Science News*, December 4, 1982. It quickly summarizes the theory, mentions Zigler's plea and his study with institutionalized children, and then tells of the latest statement issued by the American Academy of Pediatrics, again denouncing patterning (see *Pediatrics*, November 1982).

An Exposé

The final article under criticisms differs from those previously reviewed because it includes unflattering information about the staff members at the Institutes.

Philadelphia Magazine, in its April 1982 issue, printed Robin Warshaw's "The Minds of Children." It has a negative tone right from the beginning. First, Warshaw updated the Posnett case, the family that brought the Institutes so much attention in the 1960s. The child did not in fact become a "normal, active boy," as predicted in *Good Housekeeping* in 1962. The family, according to Warshaw, is bitter about being abandoned by the Institutes after the years dragged on with little improvement.

Warshaw describes Glenn Doman, who declined to be interviewed, as a "guru," "chief salesman," "of cosmic importance," "magnetic," "charismatic," and "seductive." Janet Doman, his daughter, is "intelligent but remote" and "devoted to her father." A wealthy enthusiast "bankrolled the establishment of Doman's Institutes," which Warshaw said generates $2 million in annual revenue, has a $6 million trust fund, and has purchased 52 acres for unknown purposes. Doubters and unsuccessful cases are abandoned, phony awards such as "the Brazilian Medal of Honor" are presented in military-like ceremonies. Some branches of the Institutes are in name only and maintain no staff. Children are forced to learn rote facts (as opposed to learning to be problem-solvers and independent thinkers), performances are rehearsed and staged, and the Institutes resists all verification. Parents are quoted as saying, "Doman could sell my dead grandmother a bottle of Geritol" (p. 180) and "When I got away from it, it was such a relief" (p. 184).

The Warshaw article includes two revelations that, if true, could potentially further damage the Institutes' credibility among parents and professionals. Key staff members are reportedly involved with the Church of Scientology and key staff members have purchased their college degrees.

At least as early as February 1979, according to documents obtained by Philadelphia Magazine, Janet Doman "graduated" from a Church of Scientology training session at the controversial sect's Ardmore Center (p. 180).

Her husband has also taken at least four courses, one of which was "Potential Trouble Source/Suppressive Persons Routing, Detection and Handling Course." Susan Aisen, Douglas Doman (son), and Rosalind Klein—all of whom saw Jamie and helped devise his assignments—are also reportedly involved with Scientology, as are several newcomers. At one time, until questioned by parents, "Children at the Institutes were given Scientology-oriented study materials" (p. 182); and "Glenn Doman and his Institutes have been the subjects of a glowing profile in a Scientology-oriented magazine" (p. 182). Scientology is not only a controversial cult, but eight of its high officials "were convicted of criminal activities related to a plot to infiltrate government offices and steal documents" (p. 124). "And the Church of Scientology has demonstrated an interest in the past in covertly connecting itself with various educational institutions" (p. 180).

The Institutes also sought academic recognition for its courses for parents. "Late in 1967, the Institutes tried to validate 'degrees' it bestowed for work with the brain-injured by setting up a 'graduate school'" (p. 186). The Pennsylvania State Department of Education did not approve the proposal due to inadequate faculty, incoherent course of study, and meaningless admission requirements. Nevertheless, the Institutes continued to issue Human Developmentalist certificates to staff and parents. Alden and I each have one, both in a fancy engraved diploma-like case, that qualifies us at the "Initial Parent Level." I remember Glenn Doman telling us in our private interview with him that we would learn more in that week at the Institutes than we ever would learn in a whole semester at college.

The Institutes' next attempt at educational validation of staff members can only be described by quoting at length:

> In 1975, the University of Plano [an Institutes affiliated school in Texas] board of trustees—a body which included Glenn Doman—voted to recognize certificates awarded to students from the Philadelphia Institutes as equivalent to the college's own academic degrees. This approval was granted although the recipients never studied at Plano. The Institutes' "degrees" had no accreditation and Plano itself was prohibited by Texas authorities from issuing anything higher than a bachelor's degree, since the school lacked graduate standing.
>
> A letter to college President Morris from Institutes' administrator Neil Harvey, uncovered in an investigation by the *Dallas Morning News*, acknowleged a purchase price of $100 for a Plano Doctorate, $75 for a master's, and $50 for a bachelor's degree. Recipients included Harvey himself (master's), Glenn Doman (bachelor's, master's, and doctorate), and 34 other Institutes enrollees.
>
> In mid-1975, Plano—which the Dallas newspaper described as receiving its funding from land speculation—closed for good, just a few weeks after the Institutes collected its "degrees." The degrees have never been recognized by the State of Texas certification board for colleges.
>
> ...Glenn Doman lists his doctorate from Plano and his physical therapy certificate from Penn as his two formal educational credentials. Behind the stone walls on Stenton Avenue, he is called Doctor Doman (p. 186).

When David Posnett was 17 and still seriously disabled, Doman persuaded the family to send him to the University of Plano. William Posnett, David's father, flew to Texas in response to his son's frequent calls indicating he was unhappy there. William Posnett said he found "nothing down there" and "kids left in their room all day" (p. 188).

It is interesting to note that in the 1966 paper by LeWinn, Doman, Doman, Delacato, Spitz, and Thomas in Hellmuth, Glenn Doman put "Sc.D." after his name—ten years before he even allegedly purchased the Plano degree.

I hope the preceding summaries and the following reference list will serve as a useful guide to parents and professionals seeking more information about patterning and the Institutes for the Achievement of Human Potential.

Reference List

American Academy for Cerebral Palsy, The Canadian Association for Children with Learning Disabilities, The Canadian Association for Retarded Children, The Canadian Rehabilitation Council for the Disabled, American Congress of Rehabilitation Medicine, National Association for Retarded Children, and the American Academy of Physical Medicine and Rehabilitation (1968). The Doman-Delacato treatment of neurologically handicapped children. *Journal of Pediatrics, 72,* 750-752.

American Academy of Pediatrics (1982). Policy statement: The Doman-Delacto treatment of neurologically handicapped children. *Pediatrics, 70,* 810-812.

Beck, J. (1964). Mental miracles for brain-injured children. *The Chicago Tribune Sunday Magazine,* Sept. 13, 26-44.

Beck, J. (1964). Why Johnny can read. *The Chicago Tribune Sunday Magazine,* Sept. 27, 25-32.

Bird, J. (1967). When children can't learn. *Saturday Evening Post,* July 29, 27-30, 72-74.

Briesky, W. (1974). *I think I can.* Garden City, NY: Doubleday.

Campbell, B. (1976). 60 volunteers a week aid retarded boy. *New York Times,* April 16, 1, 55.

Cohen, H. J., Birch, H. H., & Taft, L. T. (1970). Some considerations for evaluating the Doman-Delacato patterning method. *Pediatrics, 45,* 302-313.

Dart, R. (1967). *Adventures with the missing link.* Philadelphia, PA: The Institutes Press.

Delacato, C. H. (1959). *The treatment and prevention of reading problems, the neuro-psychological approach.* Springfield, IL: Thomas.

Delacato, C. H. (1963). *The diagnosis and treatment of speech and reading problems.* Springfield, IL: Thomas.

Delacato, C. H. (1966). *Neurological organization and reading.* Springfield, IL: Thomas.

Delacato, C. H. (1966). Delacato revisited. *Exceptional Children,* 33, 199-200.

Doman, G. (1964). *How to teach your baby to read.* New York: Random House.

Doman, G. (1974). *What to do about your brain-injured child or your brain damaged, mentally retarded, mentally deficient, cerebral palsied, spastic, flaccid, rigid, epileptic, autistic, athetoid, hyperactive child.* Garden City, NY: Doubleday.

Doman, G. (1979). *How to teach your baby math.* New York: Simon and Schuster.

Doman, G. (1984). *How to multiply your baby's intelligence.* New York: Doubleday.

Doman, G., Doman, J., & Aisen, S. (1985). *How to give your baby encyclopedic knowledge.* Philadelphia: The Better Baby Press.

Doman, R. J., Spitz, E. B., Zucman, E., Delacato, C., & Doman, G. (1960). Children with severe injuries, neurological organization in terms of mobility. *Journal of the American Medical Association,* 174, 257-262.

Ernst, P. (1962). Miracle in Pennsylvania. *Good Housekeeping,* Sept., 32, 34, 37-38.

Freeman, R. D. (1967). Controversy over patterning as a treatment for brain damage in children. *Journal of the American Medical Association,* 202, 385-388.

Freeman, R. D. (1967). Book review: *An investigation of the Doman-Delacato theory of neuropsychology as it applies to trainable mentally retarded children in public schools. Journal of Pediatrics,* 71, 914.

Herbert, W. (1982). Treatment for brain damage under fire. *Science News,* 122, 357.

Kerschner, J. R. (1967). *An investigation of the Doman-Delacato theory of neuropsychology as it applies to trainable mentally retarded children in public schools.* Harrisburg, PA: Bureau of Research Administration and Coordination, Department of Public Instruction, Commonwealth of Pennsylvania.

Langway, L. (1983). Bringing up superbaby. *Newsweek*, March 28, 62-68.

LeWinn, E. B. (1969). *Human neurological organization*. Springfield, IL: Thomas.

LeWinn, E. B., Doman, G., Doman, R. J., Delacato, C. H., Spitz, E., & Thomas, E. W. (1966). Neurological organization: The basis for learning. In J. Hellmuth (Ed.), *Learning disorders*. Seattle: Special Child Publications.

Maisel, A. Q. (1964). Hope for brain-injured children. *Reader's Digest*, Oct., 135-140.

Maslund, R. L. (1966). Unproven methods of treatment. *Pediatrics*, 37, 713-714.

Melton, D. (1968). *Todd*. New York: Dell.

Melton, D. (1972). *When children need help*. New York: Thomas Y. Crowell.

Melton, D. (1976). *A child called Hopeless*. New York: Prentice-Hall.

Napear, P. (1974). *Brain child, a mother's diary*. New York: Harper & Row.

Neman, R. (1975). A reply to Zigler and Seitz. *American Journal of Mental Deficiency*, 79, 493-505.

Neman, R., Roos, P., McCann, B. M., Menolascine, F. L., & Heal, L. W. (1975). An experimental evaluation of sensorimotor patterning used with mentally retarded children. *American Journal of Mental Deficiency*, 79, 372-384.

Pettay, H. (1984). Therapy plan turns into one family's adventure. *The York Weekly*, March 12, 1, 24-25.

Pieper, E. (n.d.). *Sticks and stones: The story of a loving child*. Syracuse: Human Policy Press.

Robbins, M. P. (1966). A study of the validity of Delacato's theory of neurological organization. *Exceptional Children*, 32, 517-523.

Robbins, M. P. (1966). A reply. *Exceptional Children*, 33, 200-201.

Robbins, M. P., & Glass, G. V. (1969). Test of the Doman-Delacato rationale with retarded readers. *Journal of the American Medical Association*, 202, 389-393.

Thomas, E. W. (1969). *Brain injured children, with special reference to Doman-Delacato methods of treatment.* Springfield, IL: C. C. Thomas.

Veras, R., with Melton, D. (1975). *Children of dreams, children of hope.* Chicago: Henry Regnery Company.

Warshaw, R. (1982). The minds of children. *Philadelphia Magazine,* April, 120-124, 180-189.

Winn, J. (1983). Boosting baby's IQ. *Saturday Evening Post,* Nov., 46-47, 104-105.

Wolf, J. M. (1968). *Temple Fay, progenitor of the Doman-Delacato procedures.* Springfield, IL: Thomas.

Zigler, E. (1981). A plea to end the use of the patterning treatment for retarded children. *American Journal of Orthopsychiatry,* 51, 388-390.

Zigler, E., & Seitz, V. (1975). On "An experimental evaluation of sensorimotor patterning": A critique. *American Journal of Mental Deficiency,* 79, 483-492.

Zigler, E., & Sparrow, S. (1978). Evaluation of a patterning treatment for retarded children. *Pediatrics,* 62, 137-150.